General Hospital Care for People with Learning Disabilities

Lynn Hannon

Julie Clift

WILEY-BLACKWELL

A John Wiley & Sons, Ltd., Publication

This edition first published 2011
© 2011 Blackwell Publishing Ltd

Blackwell Publishing was acquired by John Wiley & Sons in February 2007. Blackwell's publishing programme has been merged with Wiley's global Scientific, Technical, and Medical business to form Wiley-Blackwell.

Registered office
John Wiley & Sons Ltd, The Atrium, Southern Gate, Chichester, West Sussex, PO19 8SQ, United Kingdom

Editorial offices
9600 Garsington Road, Oxford, OX4 2DQ, United Kingdom
2121 State Avenue, Ames, Iowa 50014-8300, USA

For details of our global editorial offices, for customer services and for information about how to apply for permission to reuse the copyright material in this book please see our website at www.wiley.com/wiley-blackwell.

Library of Congress Cataloging-in-Publication Data

Hannon, Lynn.
   General hospital care for people with learning disabilities / Lynn Hannon, Julie Clift.
      p. ; cm.
   Includes bibliographical references and index.
   ISBN 978-1-4051-8563-9 (pbk. : alk. paper)   1. Learning disabled–Hospital care.
2. Learning disabilities–Nursing.   I. Clift, Julie.   II. Title.
   [DNLM: 1. Learning Disorders–nursing. 2. Hospitalization. WY 160 H2368g 2011]
   RC394.L37H36 2011
   362.196′85889–dc22

                                                                  2010016797

A catalogue record for this book is available from the British Library.

Set in 10/12 pt Times by Aptara® Inc., New Delhi, India
Printed and bound in Malaysia by Vivar Printing Sdn Bhd

1   2011

General Hospital
Learning Disabilities

Contents

Preface

This book is about general hospital care for people with a learning disability. It explores the nature of learning disability and highlights how to identify and meet the particular health needs of people with a learning disability.

The book takes the reader through all the key factors in the health care process from pre-admission assessment and identification of health needs, person-centred care planning, leading to successful treatment interventions and planned discharge.

It focuses on the key areas of communication, behaviour and consent, and highlights how multidisciplinary approaches can contribute to successful outcomes for everyone involved.

The Department of Health (1999, 2001), National Health Service Executive (NHSE 1998) and Mencap (1998), all have reported that people with learning disabilities have increased health needs to the general population, yet these needs are often poorly met, and people experience difficulties in accessing appropriate services.

The NHSE (1998) recommended that 'Mainstream National Health Services need to become more responsive to the special circumstances and needs of people with learning disabilities'.

It is hoped that this book will serve as a comprehensive resource for health care professionals working in general hospital settings, who may come into contact with people with a learning disability in the course of their working life, providing information, practical examples and good practice guidance to enable them to understand and meet the health needs of people with a learning disability.

The first chapter explores the nature of learning disability and the specific health care needs of people with a learning disability. It considers the key factors that influence the health care process, and stresses the importance of person-centred approaches.

The book then takes the reader through the patient journey and the process of health care, through pre-admission assessment, care planning, intervention and treatment, liaison and discharge planning.

This is followed by chapters on the key aspects of communication, behaviour management and the often difficult area of consent.

The book finishes with a chapter exploring the ethical and political aspects of health care, abuse issues and safeguarding of people with a learning disability, the value of multidisciplinary approaches and good practice benchmarks.

The book is relevant to the care of both children and adults with a learning disability and case vignettes are used throughout to illustrate situations.

The use of case studies throughout this book are intended to help illustrate examples of situations explored in main text and are not intended to be a template for action in similar situations.

This book also includes reference to a research project looking at pre-admission assessment for people with a learning disability conducted by one of the authors.

REFERENCES

Department of Health (1999) *Facing the Facts*. HMSO, London.
Department of Health (2001) *Valuing People*. HMSO, London.
Mencap (1998) *Health for All*. Mencap, London.
NHS Executive (1998) *Signposts for Success*. HMSO, London.

Acknowledgements

First and foremost, we acknowledge the journey we have made together in writing this book. As experienced nurses, but novice authors, it has been a real voyage of discovery and adventure. We feel that we have risen to the challenge, learning much along the way, and we are proud of our achievement in completing this book.

This book and the case studies used for illustration are based on our real-life experiences. We would like to express our thanks and appreciation to all the individuals who have been willing to share their stories with us and who have helped us along the way.

We value the support of our families and friends, for putting up with the long working days and late nights, and for keeping us going when times were tough. We also appreciate the encouragement and support we have received from our academic and work colleagues in hospital and community-based services.

Particular thanks must go to Bev French, MSc Course Leader at University of Central Lancashire (UCLAN), for her encouragement and support with developing the early ideas and the pre-admission assessment research project. Special thanks also go to the Florence Nightingale Foundation for their award of a Travel Scholarship funded by the Sandra Charitable Trust to enable study and development of the original research.

Our colleagues at East Lancashire Hospitals Trust have provided great support in developing the Acute Liaison Nurse role, and have also embraced the challenge of changing their practice in meeting the health needs of people with learning disabilities. In particular, Brigid Reid, Nurse Consultant and Head of Patient Experience, who brought her enthusiasm for the work we were doing and said, 'If we can get it right for people with a learning disability we can get it right for everybody.'

Our thanks go to Mencap for permission to use their images, Rick Robson and A2A for permission to reproduce materials, and to the Makaton Charity for permission to reproduce their symbols. We also thank our publishers who gave great support and advice to us as novice authors.

Our most grateful thanks and respect go to all the people with learning disabilities and their families, who we have worked with over many years and who have taught us so much and inspired our practice.

This book is particularly dedicated to the memory of Martin, Emma, Mark, Ted, Tom and Warren, the six people with a learning disability whose stories provided us all with so many valuable lessons to be learned. We hope this book will contribute to enabling health care staff working in general hospitals to provide high-quality and effective care to all people with a learning disability in the future.

1 Understanding Learning Disability

INTRODUCTION

This book is designed to provide a framework of good practice guidance to support health care professionals working in general hospital services to provide care to people with a learning disability. This first chapter provides an introduction to the nature of learning disability and insight into what this means for the person. It explores how to establish if your patient has a learning disability, and the perceptions and attitudes of health care professionals towards people with a learning disability. The chapter then continues to summarise what the current evidence base says about how to identify and meet the health needs of people with a learning disability, including factors and barriers that influence the health care process and how to overcome these. The needs of families and carers are highlighted and the important role they have to play in the process. The chapter concludes with an introduction to the person-centred approaches that are a central aspect of learning disability practice.

We do not always know who is disabled. Many people associate disability with wheelchair use, yet less than 5% of disabled people use a wheelchair. Anyone who meets the following definition from the Disability Discrimination Act (DDA) (Department of Health 1995b) is considered to be disabled:

> Someone with a *physical* or *mental impairment* which has a *substantial* and *long-term* adverse effect on their ability to carry out normal *day to day activities*.

This includes *physical impairments* to senses such as sight and hearing, and *mental impairments* such as learning disabilities and mental illness. Conditions covered may include things such as severe depression, diabetes, dyslexia, epilepsy and arthritis.

Substantial includes:

- Inability to see moving traffic clearly enough to cross a road safely
- Inability to turn taps or knobs
- Inability to remember and relay a simple message correctly

Long-term means that the effects have lasted, or are expected to last 12 months or more.

Day-to-day activities include mobility, manual dexterity, physical coordination, continence, ability to lift, speech, hearing, eyesight, memory and recognising physical danger.

Considering the Disability Discrimination Act definition of disability, it is clear that a wide range of people and health conditions could be incorporated within this.

General Hospital Care for People with Learning Disabilities, First Edition by Lynn Hannon and Julie Clift
© 2011 Blackwell Publishing Ltd

The new Equality Act 2010 will come into force in October 2010. The Act brings disability, sex, race and other grounds of discrimination within one piece of legislation, and also makes changes to the law. Further information about the Act can be found at: http://www.equalities.gov.uk/equality_act_2010.aspx

DEFINITIONS AND CAUSES OF A LEARNING DISABILITY

Definitions

A learning disability is a lifelong condition, which has its beginning before, during or after birth, or as a result of injury to the brain before the age of 18, which affects an individual's ability to learn, communicate or do everyday things. A learning disability is not an illness, and whilst the condition cannot be 'cured', it is possible for an individual with a learning disability to develop new skills and progress.

A learning disability should not be confused with educational 'learning difficulties' such as dyslexia, and hyperactive disorders, or mental illness, which are other conditions, not covered within this book. People who acquire brain injuries after the age of 18 are not normally considered to have a learning disability, as the injury has occurred after the brain was fully developed.

Mackenzie (2005), cited in Grant et al. (2005, p. 49), explains that 'the international *Classification of Mental and Behavioural Disorders* (ICD-10) (World Health Organisation 1992) and the *Diagnostic and Statistical Manual of Mental Disorders* (DSM-IV) (American Psychiatric Association 1994) are the main classification systems currently in use'. ICD is the system used in the UK. Both these systems use the term 'mental retardation' and this equates to learning disability. Whilst the term 'mental retardation' may be defined in the ICD, it is however unacceptable for use in clinical practice.

Mackenzie outlines the following (broadly similar) ICD and DSM definitions of learning disability:

DSM-IV definition

1. Significantly subaverage intellectual functioning: an intelligence quotient (IQ) of approximately 70 or below on an individually administered IQ test (for infants, a clinical judgement of significantly subaverage intellectual functioning).
2. Concurrent deficits or impairments in present adaptive functioning (i.e. the person's effectiveness in meeting the standards expected for his or her age by his or her cultural group) in at least two of the following areas: communication, self-care, home living, social/interpersonal skills, use of community resources, self-direction, functional academic skills, work, leisure, health and safety.
3. The onset is before 18 years of age.

ICD-10 definition

Mental retardation is a condition of arrested or incomplete development of mind, which is characterised by impairment of skills manifested during the developmental period, which contribute to the overall level of intelligence, i.e. cognitive, language, motor and social abilities.

Mackenzie also explains that 'each is based on the presence of impairments in adaptive function in association with low intelligence quotient (IQ)'.

You may have heard of a variety of different terms used to describe someone with a learning disability, many of them are now considered to be inappropriate, and some are actually offensive and should never be used.

Reflective Learning Point:

Think about all the terms you may have heard to define a learning disability and how they would sound to a person with a learning disability and their family.

Mackenzie (2005), cited in Grant et al. (2005), continues to describe the following World Health Organisation (1980) definitions:

- Impairment – Any loss or abnormality of physical or psychological function
- Disability – Interference with activities of the whole person (usually described in learning disability practice as activities of daily living)
- Handicap – The social disadvantage to an individual as a result of impairment or a disability

The Mental Health Act (Department of Health 1983) uses the term 'mental impairment', and the term 'mental handicap' may still be used, though this is not considered acceptable any more. All these terms can be seen to represent what people may consider as features of a disability. A social model of disability, as opposed to a medical model, identifies attitudes and environment as being major causes of disability, and not the personal abilities of the people involved. The medical model focuses on the clinical aspects of the condition and how it is treated, and not necessarily the impact on the person.

The Department of Health (2001a) report 'Valuing People' defines a learning disability as having the following characteristics:

- A significantly reduced ability to understand new or complex information, to learn new skills (impairment of intelligence)
- A reduced ability to cope independently (impaired social functioning)
- Started before adulthood (usually considered to be age 18), with a lasting effect on development

Each individual goes through a comprehensive process of assessment before a diagnosis of learning disability can be confirmed. A syndrome is the medical term for a recognised set of clinical features which commonly occur together. Some syndromes (e.g. Down's syndrome) are named after the person who first described them or others after a particular feature of the syndrome.

Mackenzie (2005) (cited in Grant et al. 2005, p. 49) outlines that 'the term "special needs" refers to children who have been given a Statement of special educational needs by their local education authority. The educational category of severe learning difficulties corresponds more closely with learning disabilities as used in health settings'.

Intelligence is formally measured through a cognitive assessment by a qualified clinical psychologist, who gives people an IQ score. The Royal College of Nursing (2006) explains how IQ range is naturally distributed in the population and the average IQ (mean score) is 100,

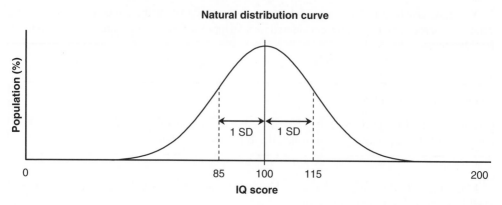

Fig. 1.1 Natural distribution of IQ. Adapted from Grant et al. (2005). Reproduced with the kind permission of Open University Press. All rights reserved.

with a standard deviation range of 15 points on either side. Therefore, anyone with an IQ score between 85 and 115 is said to be of average intelligence (Fig. 1.1).

The range of 1 standard deviation above or below the mean represents 68% of the population. Another 28% of the population has an IQ score within 2 standard deviations of the mean (14% above and 14% below), leaving a small number of individuals (2%) at either end of the scale outside of 2 standard deviations of the mean.

The range of IQ distribution in the population is illustrated in Table 1.1.

From this table we can see that approximately 2% of the population can be considered to have a learning disability.

Impairment of intelligence can be presented at different levels and the British Psychological Society (2000) explains that:

- People with an IQ of 55–69 can be said to have a *significant* impairment in intellectual functioning.
- People with an IQ of below 55 can be said to have a *severe* impairment in intellectual functioning.

IQ tests are not routinely carried out for all people with a learning disability, so this information may not be available for the people that you see. A referral can be made when a need to measure intelligence is identified, for example when capacity to consent issues arises.

The term 'mild learning disability' may be used to describe a *significant* impairment, and the terms 'moderate, severe or profound' may be used to describe a *severe* impairment in intellectual functioning. The term 'intellectual disability' is commonly used in other countries. Some people with an IQ in the range 70–85 can find that their learning impairment is often not diagnosed at an early age, and they are not able to access services designed for people with significant or severe impairments.

Table 1.1 The range of IQ distribution in the population

IQ range	55–70 and below	71–85	86–100	101–115	116–130	131–145 and above
Population (%)	2	14	34	34	14	2

Prevalence

Mencap (2002) reported, 'There are about 1.5 million people with a mild or moderate learning disability, and an estimated 210,000 individuals with severe or profound and multiple learning disabilities currently living in the United Kingdom'.

Michaels (2008, p. 14) reported that 'estimates of the prevalence of learning disability vary reflecting differences in definition. Department of Health figures suggest that about 1.5 million people (around 2.5% of the UK population) have a learning disability'. He also cited Emerson and Hatton (2004), who suggest that '3% of children and 2% of adults fall into the category overall. Of these, 1.2 million people have mild-moderate learning disability and around 210,000 (about one third of 1%) have severe and profound learning disabilities. This latter group includes 65,000 children and young people, 120,000 adults of working age and 25,000 older people'.

Michaels (2008) continues to explain that:

> The prevalence of learning disability in the general population is expected to rise by around 1% per annum for the next 10 years and to grow overall by over 10% by 2020. It is also expected that there will be a growth in the complexity of disabilities. This is attributable to improvements in maternal and neonatal care and improvements in general health care for adults which lead to increased life expectancy. Increasing use of alcohol in the UK and rates of unplanned teenage pregnancy are also expected to contribute to increases in the prevalence of foetal alcohol syndrome (which is a specific syndrome with associated learning disability as a clinical feature). In addition, there are increases anticipated in the proportion of younger English adults from South Asian minority ethnic communities where the prevalence of learning disability is higher.

It is clear then that a significant number of individuals can be affected by a learning disability. Severe learning disability is more easily recognised and diagnosed and is relatively evenly spread in the population. Accurate reporting of mild to moderate levels of learning disability is more difficult, with a number of people not diagnosed until adulthood when they are coming into contact with various health or social services. Some people are not correctly diagnosed at all and may even be given alternative labels such as a mental health diagnosis.

Some areas of the UK have higher levels of people with a learning disability in their community due to the previous existence of a long-stay learning disability hospital in the area. People were often resettled from the hospital to the local community instead of returning to the place they had been admitted from.

Causes and diagnosis

As outlined previously, a learning disability is a lifelong condition, which has its beginning before, during or after birth, or as a result of injury to the brain before the age of 18.

The main causes of learning disability can be considered as follows:

- *Before birth*: For example, genetic conditions such as Down's syndrome, metabolic disorders and maternal infections
- *During birth*: For example, lack of oxygen and trauma
- *After birth and before age of 18*: For example, accidents causing brain injury and infections

The cause does not always give an indication of the level of learning disability; for example, people with Down's syndrome can range in ability levels from mild to severe impairment. The level of disability and the subsequent impact on the ability of the person can vary across a wide range, from people who can live quite independently with minimal support to people who need full nursing care and are completely reliant on others.

Reflective Learning Point:

Look at the following pictures – Who do you think has a learning disability?

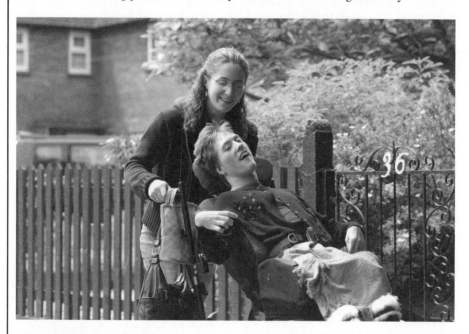

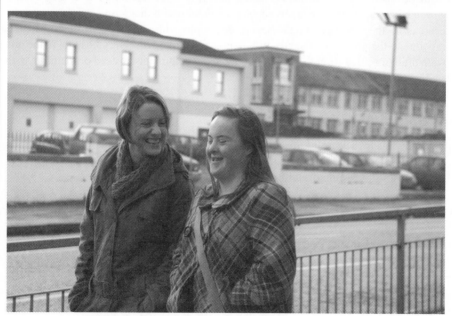

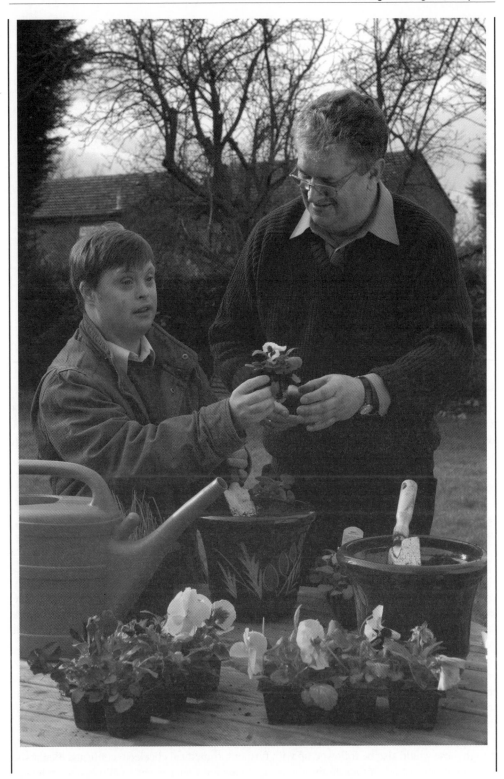

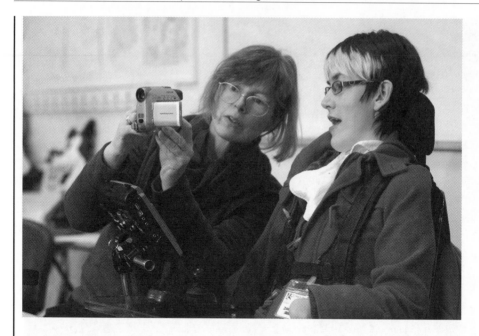

Photo: Mencap (2009).

The answer is we do not know for sure, but we do make assumptions based on what we see.

Although it is not possible to explore the full range of learning disability conditions in detail within this book, there are numerous publications available through your local health library for anyone interested in condition-related information. Further information about specific health needs associated with a learning disability is outlined later in this chapter.

Mackenzie (2005), cited in Grant et al. (2005, p. 48), outlines the 'bio-psycho-social' model now taught in medical schools:

> This model places the patient (as a unique individual with biological, psychological and social needs) at the centre of their interaction with health services. It is within this framework that the process of diagnosis and assessment of the health needs of an individual with learning disabilities and the planning of health services to meet their needs should take place.

She continues to explain (cited in Grant et al. 2005, p. 55) that 'in 80% of people with severe learning disabilities, a specific bio-medical cause can be diagnosed'. This also demonstrates that there are a number of people (20%) with a learning disability where the exact cause cannot be defined.

The process of diagnosis begins with some routine screening tests that are offered during pregnancy (e.g. for Down's syndrome). Where there is a family history of a particular genetic condition, specific screening can also take place for this. Other screening tests are carried out soon after a child is born (e.g. a heel prick blood test for phenylketonuria), which can lead to successful treatment and prevention of a learning disability developing.

Some conditions have clearly recognisable clinical features that can be identified at birth, though these would also be followed up with further bio-medical checks to confirm a diagnosis. Other diagnoses of a learning disability are not made until later when a child is not achieving developmental milestones as expected, and this is investigated further. The assessment and diagnosis process also helps to identify any associated physical or developmental needs that may require specific treatment. Early intervention for these now can improve long-term health outcomes for the individual.

Some learning disability conditions have specific health problems associated with them, and the diagnosis should help with identifying and planning to meet these health needs. Mackenzie (cited in Grant et al. 2005, p. 63) outlines an example of the health problems known to be associated with Down's syndrome:

- Congenital heart defects
- Respiratory infections
- Hearing and visual impairments
- Hypothyroidism
- Skin problems
- Gum disease and tooth loss
- Obesity
- Depression
- Alzheimer's disease (early onset)

This example illustrates the multiple and complex health needs associated with one of the most commonly recognised learning disability conditions. Learning Disability Nurses have a good understanding of the health needs of people with a learning disability and can provide information and valuable support to health care professionals in general hospital settings.

A diagnosis of a learning disability has a great impact on a family, especially where there has been no indication during a pregnancy to cause any concern. Parents of a child with a learning disability often look for a diagnosis to explain how this has occurred, and also to help them to come to terms with what the impact will be on their present and future lives. This can be a very difficult time, and sensitive support from health care professionals can be very reassuring. It is also important to consider referral for genetic counselling where appropriate – though this is too detailed a topic to explore further within this book.

HOW TO ESTABLISH IF YOUR PATIENT HAS A LEARNING DISABILITY

You cannot always tell just by looking at someone if they have a learning disability. Sometimes it is obvious when a person has a recognisable condition (e.g. Down's syndrome) or some physical disabilities, but most of the time it is not so easy to identify. It can be particularly difficult for health care professionals to judge levels of functioning when people present as being more able and capable than they actually are.

In order to establish if your patient has a learning disability, you will need to investigate the following key points:

- *Is there a diagnosis of learning disability?* This may be a more obvious condition such as Down's syndrome, or conditions such as autism, or Prader–Willi syndrome. Is anything written in their medical records?
- *Do they access services that support people with a learning disability?* Day services, social services, special hospitals.

- *Where do they live?* Do they have support in the home or do they live in a supported living environment?
- *Did the person go to a special school, or receive support to attend a mainstream school?*
- *Do they have support from learning disability services?* This could be a consultant psychiatrist, community nurse, social worker, speech and language therapist, psychologist.
- *Can the person read and write?*
- *Check any records* you may have access to for any previous reference to a learning disability.

Some behavioural indicators may be:

- Slow or confused response to questioning
- Difficulty retaining personal information, details or events
- Immature behaviour
- Inappropriate social behaviour, for example over familiarity

Some communication indicators may be:

- Unclear in relaying personal information
- Unable to tell you who they are and what is wrong with them
- Unclear about time of day, date or place
- Echolalic – repeats back to you what you have said
  (See also further information in Chapter 3.)

People who have attained General Certificate of Secondary Education (GCSE) (or equivalent) at a–c level, drive a car, or attended mainstream school without support would not usually be considered to have a learning disability. However, this is just a guide and there may be exceptions. If you are unclear but suspect that the person has a learning disability and would benefit from support during the admission, information could be obtained from your local Social Services Department or Community Learning Disability Team.

PERCEPTIONS AND ATTITUDES TOWARDS PEOPLE WITH A LEARNING DISABILITY

Health care professionals may work in general hospital services for many years without having to work with people with a learning disability. A lack of exposure can lead to an associated lack of awareness or understanding of the health needs of people with a learning disability, creating a perception that working with them will be a difficult or unpleasant experience.

Perception can be explained as the process we use to collect, interpret and comprehend information from the world around us by means of our senses. We then use this information to recognise what will happen in a particular situation. Some people may be described as very perceptive because they are able to reach this conclusion quickly. An attitude can be described as your point of view or position on something, the way you think and feel about something. Attitudes are created from your perception, whether this is based on fact or otherwise, and both your perception and attitude can create a barrier between the health care professional and a person with a learning disability before you even meet them.

Health care professionals' initial perception of people with a learning disability is commonly founded on stereotypes or information provided by other people rather than based on their own experiences. This information is often exaggerated and is usually describing negative reports of the experiences of other people.

Reflective Learning Point:

Describe to a colleague how you would feel now if you were informed that the next patient you were to see has a learning disability.

- What would your initial thoughts be?
- What would you expect the person to be like?

A number of different studies have considered the attitudes of health care professionals towards people with learning disabilities. Biley (1994) reported that nurses' negative attitudes towards people with disabilities admitted to acute hospital settings could make for a traumatic stay. She highlighted a general lack of awareness of the needs of patients with a physical disability and also that 'although differing impairments have different disabling effects, most people with a disability are handicapped primarily by negative attitudes and the limited range of choices available to them'.

Shanley and Guest (1995) describe the stigmatisation of people with learning disabilities as 'a barrier to good nursing care'. They suggested that 'the educational preparation of general nurses must facilitate greater awareness of stigmatised groups'. This is a point that is often raised and yet has not been addressed fully by the training establishments and incorporated enough into basic training programmes for health care professionals.

The influences of contact, and graduate/non-graduate status, on the attitudes of nurses in a general hospital towards people with learning disabilities were explored by Slevin and Sines (1996). They reported that 'attitudes held were more negative than would be expected from those in a caring profession'. The graduate nurses were found to be more positive than non-graduate nurses are. Nurses in the sample who had experienced higher amounts of contact with people with a learning disability were found to have more positive attitudes. This is consistent with the general lack of confidence of hospital staff in working with people with a learning disability that is shown in the summary of the evidence base later in this chapter, and also with the evidence that attitudes of health care professionals become more positive, the more time they spend with people with a learning disability.

Hannon (2003) found that whilst experience is identified in the evidence base as an influencing factor on attitudes, a positive attitude was seen in a hospital staff who had only been qualified for 2 years, and had only minimal previous contact with people with a learning disability. All hospital staff in the study felt they treated everyone the same, and the experiences of people with a learning disability in this research project were more positive than expected, with service users all reporting that they felt that they were treated the same as everyone else. It was found that what tended to stick in the mind are difficult situations and that this needs to be balanced out with positive experiences. Hospital staff were pleasantly surprised to meet people that they actually enjoyed having on the ward. Initial fear about caring for the person was changed in the light of their experience. This evidence of a more positive attitude after contact supports previous research (Slevin & Sines 1996).

Hannon also noted that hospital staff were more confident with more able people but less so where there were behavioural or communication problems, or other complex needs. The hospital staff expressed that they felt they had a lack of experience, training and preparation to enable them to care effectively for this client group. They felt that they had a lack of information about learning disability and felt that it should be included within pre-registration education programmes.

The findings from this study agree with a review of other available research by Fitzsimmons and Barr (1997), who found a number of variables that influenced attitudes including the perceived severity of disability, confusion about the definition of a learning disability, behaviour, communication, and poor preparation and training. Melville et al. (2007) (cited in Michael 2008, p. 35) assessed the training needs of 210 practice nurses and delivered a bespoke training package that had a significant impact on knowledge and practice. People with a learning disability are also involved in some areas in providing this training themselves (e.g. at St Georges Hospital Medical School) with very positive feedback.

The following two case studies illustrate how the perceptions and attitudes of health care professionals were changed following their experience of caring for someone with a learning disability in hospital. The figures in brackets are references to interview transcripts recorded during the (Hannon) research project.

Understanding Learning Disability Case Study 1 – Steven

Steven is 17 years old and was admitted to hospital for the first time. He has a mild learning disability, minor communication difficulties, but no behaviour problems. He is fully independent with personal care, and did not need anyone to stay with him. Steven is quite a shy person. He was admitted to an adult ward, and was visited by his consultant paediatrician.

Steven lives with his father, who also has a mild learning disability. He stayed with Steven during admission process and then left. He was concerned to find out what was wrong with Steven, but not about the admission. [19.422] '(Community Learning Disability (LD) Nurse) helped a lot because she explained that he had never been in before and had a word with the nurse'.

The Community Learning Disability Nurse was present for the admission. She has 18 years' experience, but has known Steven only for 3 months. She had previous experience of supporting people with learning disabilities in hospital. The hospital staff caring for Steven was a qualified nurse with 30 years' experience, including previous experience working with people with learning disabilities in hospital.

Steven stayed in the main ward. He would have preferred a single room but there was not one available. He did not like listening to another patient vomiting, and was distracted by other patients moving around when he was trying to sleep. He felt hungry because he could not eat prior to investigation.

Following pre-admission assessment, the community nurse had liaised with hospital staff to discuss Steven's fear of needles. He had blood samples taken through the sensitive approach of hospital staff, and support of his community nurse. What helped Steven was [20.584–592] 'I would need the things explained to me, yes, so I don't get confused, so they can tell me what they were going to do. So they didn't do it behind my back, so they got me prepared for it'.

Father appreciated support from the community nurse and felt that carers do not get the same response as another professional. [19.544–548] 'I still say with (community nurse) putting them in the picture it helped. It is better than me talking. Somebody speaking up and telling them before they do anything'.

Meeting Steven positively influenced the attitude of the hospital staff. [18.32–33] 'Unfortunately people always have a perception about somebody with a learning disability and maybe you think they are going to be very noisy and very destructive. I think that is probably general. He wasn't like that at all, he was very shy, a very quiet person'.

Steven felt that hospital staff overprotected him. Being on an adult ward could have influenced this, or perhaps it reflects the view that people with a learning disability are 'perpetual children' and need to be cared for. His father thought hospital staff were just caring. The community nurse felt that hospital staff [17.93] 'were very friendly, but they were friendly in a way that they were talking to a child, and at 17 he is a young man'.

The researcher noted a point made by hospital staff about communication. [18.147–155] 'Well if it's more of a language barrier we get interpreters. If it's deaf and dumb there are people we can get to do sign language. We have access to hearing facilities and Braille'. When the researcher mentioned that people with learning disabilities use a communication system called Makaton, hospital staff replied, [18.161] 'We wouldn't have a clue what Makaton is'. *(See Chapter 3 for information about Makaton.)*

The community nurse felt she had a positive opportunity to promote her role. [17.146] 'I felt valued as a fellow practitioner and I felt valued that the contribution that I had for this young man's admission and discharge'. Everyone involved saw the admission as successful.

Understanding Learning Disability Case Study 2 – Lucy

Lucy is a 47-year-old woman with a mild to moderate learning disability. She is friendly and talkative, and understands everything said to her if people talk slowly. She is very capable and needs minimal help with personal care. She does not have any behaviour problems. Lucy did not need anyone to stay with her, and had regular visits from people who know her.

Her carer was a social service staff with 8 years' experience, but was not a regular carer for Lucy. She completed the pre-admission assessment but had no involvement in the admission. The hospital staff involved with the initial admission had 25 years' nursing experience, and previous experience of working with people with a learning disability in hospital. She had also worked as a cadet nurse at a local learning disability hospital. The named nurse during admission had been qualified for 2 years and had met only a handful of people with a learning disability. Lucy's community nurse has 24 years' experience and has known her for 15 years.

Lucy reported that she had [11.18] 'a nice welcome' and that [11.28] 'they were all right with me'. She was pleased that hospital staff showed her around the ward and took time to explain things. She was able to correct the spelling of her surname on her medical records. Hospital staff said, [10.41] 'She was quite a nice lady', [12.44] 'She settled in really well, she was a really nice and friendly person', and [10.62] 'I would like to say Lucy was treated the same as other people, just taking a little bit more thought about her special needs'.

Hospital staff knew they needed to present information in a way she could understand. [12.151] 'We needed to know about the reading and writing, about speaking slowly and clearly'. They showed good awareness of the potential to over-protect, [12.47] 'I was trying not to be patronising; I don't want her to think I am talking down to her'.

Lucy wakes early in the morning and enjoys a cup of tea then when at home. Hospital staff were able to continue this during her admission. Her community nurse said, [9.129] 'Little things, but it means a lot to Lucy and the way she lives'. Hospital staff also liaised well with her carers to ensure support at discharge.

Lucy said, [11.53] 'The nurses and doctors were very kind to me', [11.214] 'Talked to you nicely, they don't shout they talk, they are not nasty, they tell you in front of your face what's going on'. She commented that [11.130–132] 'I couldn't understand the doctors because they were talking too fast'. Lucy appreciated the support of her community nurse at admission, [11.298–305] 'She just gave me a little talk, very nice and kind, and she tells you what's going on and everything. I was all right after that'. Her community nurse felt, [9.114] 'They were really good with her, fantastic'.

One hospital staff said, [12.112] 'You think it's going to be hard work, it's going to be trouble, but it was completely the opposite'. Another hospital staff felt, [10.193] 'For the ward I think it is probably a good experience for the ward. Like you say the more you come into contact with people with disabilities then the better it is for you'. One hospital staff thought 'mentoring' was a good approach to improve confidence, [15.105] 'Working with people that are confident so they can see it is not quite as difficult as they imagined'.

Whilst none of the hospital staff involved were aware of Community Learning Disability Services, they were all very positive about the input from Community Learning Disability Nurses. Everyone involved saw the admission as successful.

These two case studies illustrate that the perception of the hospital staff involved was that the admission would be problematic and the person may be difficult to work with, and that this perception was changed in the light of their positive experience. It was clear that the preparation for admission and support provided by carers and the Community Learning Disability Nurse enabled the admission to be successful. (*Further information about the pre-admission assessment process is outlined in Chapter 2.*)

It is important to highlight the issue of 'diagnostic overshadowing'. Mencap (2004, p. 13) outlines that 'Many families of people with a learning disability report that some doctors look at their son or daughter and – consciously or unconsciously – believe their health problem is as a result of the learning disability and that not much can be done about it. This is a dangerous assumption to make: it can lead to undiagnosed or misdiagnosed conditions. It is sometimes called "diagnostic overshadowing" and is described as "dismissing changes in behaviour, personality or ability that would be taken very seriously in a person without a learning disability"'.

The following case study highlights the issue of diagnostic overshadowing and the actual impact on an individual.

Understanding Learning Disability Case Study 3 – Laura's story

'Laura was a very active, independent woman when I first knew her. That all changed when she went into hospital last year for an emergency operation. When I went in to visit Laura after her operation, I wasn't surprised at first that she wasn't talking at all. She'd been through a major operation and I thought she must still be in recovery. I expected the old Laura to be back before long. But over the following two days I got more and more worried because she wasn't improving at all. And she didn't say a word, no matter how much I chatted to her. On the third day I asked one of the nurses if she knew why Laura wasn't speaking. She looked surprised and said, "Can she speak?" I told her that Laura could speak as well as anybody else. There was no reason for anybody to assume otherwise.

I went back in to see Laura and I offered her a pen and paper, thinking that she might be able to communicate with me that way. Laura couldn't even hold the pen. When I saw the pen roll onto the floor, I suddenly thought, oh my God, she's had a stroke. Two days later, the doctors confirmed that Laura had suffered a stroke during her operation.'

Mencap (2004), *Treat Me Right.*

Reflective Learning Point:

How would you have noticed this if you had been caring for Laura? What would help you to avoid this happening again?

HEALTH NEEDS OF PEOPLE WITH A LEARNING DISABILITY

The majority of people with a learning disability have always lived in the family home; however, over the past 20–30 years there has been a significant shift in government policy towards reducing the number of people with a learning disability living in long-stay hospitals, the majority of which have now been closed. These institutional forms of care have been replaced by residential and supported housing schemes in the community and many people also live independently in their own homes.

Mencap (2004) reported that:

> Thirty years ago 60,000 people with a learning disability lived in long stay hospitals. It was seen as the hospital's responsibility to meet their health needs. These hospitals were regarded as specialist learning disability services. As a result mainstream health services did not see (and some still do not see) people with a learning disability as being their responsibility.

The health needs of people with a learning disability were previously met within the long-stay hospitals, and people did not often access general health services. Changing care practices and the emergence of community-based care have presented general hospital services with a new challenge.

Mencap (2002) suggest that:

> Such a change in policy has been a major factor in bringing greater independence, freedom and choice to the lives of people with a learning disability, enabling them to make active, valued contributions to their communities. For such individuals any understanding of their own 'quality of life' is much the same as that of other members of the community: they value the control they have over their lives, and they reflect their own individual characters, dispositions and plans by making independent choices.

They continue to state that:

> People with learning disabilities have the same rights as any other individual to inclusion and participation in all the different levels of society. They are entitled to the provision of health care resources and treatment that meet their needs. This is so because people with a learning disability are individuals with *rights* that should enable them to pursue the same set of goals and aspirations as all other members of the community. Their rights and equal value in society should never be undermined by the nature of their disability. (Mencap 2002)

Caring for people with a learning disability in general hospitals can present a challenge even to experienced health care professionals. Learning disability covers a wide and complex range of clinical features and associated conditions, and each person has an entirely individual set of needs. The Royal College of Physicians (1998) described 'disability' as 'a disabled person's encounter with daily living, the environment and society'. They acknowledge that whilst some people may be independent at home, a hospital environment might prove to be disabling.

Summary of current evidence base

The Department of Health (1999, 2001a) and Mencap (1998, 2004, 2007) have all reported that people with a learning disability have increased health needs than the general population, yet these needs are often poorly met and people experience difficulties in accessing appropriate services. General hospital services show a wide variation in effectiveness of health care provision. There are a number of variables relating to the service user, the general hospital staff, and the organisation, which influence the success of the health care process.

Service user variables relating to people with a learning disability include:

- Difficulty in identifying and meeting their own health needs
- Difficulties in communicating – especially to explain when they do not feel well or to indicate pain
- A lack of awareness of the range of health services available
- A lack of understanding of why they need a particular health intervention – which may lead to a failure to attend appointments
- Difficulties in accessing appropriate services – either physical access or support needed to attend health appointments

In addition, many people with a learning disability are unemployed or living within lower socio-economic groups, and a higher level of ill health is associated with people within these groups.

The current evidence base highlights a number of key variables relating to general hospital staff and the organisation that influence access to general hospital services including:

- Hospital staff not understanding the specific health needs of people with a learning disability
- Problems with communication and behaviour – and a lack of knowledge of how to deal with these
- Under-/overprotectiveness
- Carers having to stay with people to provide basic care
- Negative attitudes and a lack of confidence of hospital staff working with people with a learning disability
- A lack of learning disability-specific training included within pre- and post-registration training for health care professionals

Table 1.2 Strength of evidence

Type	Strength of evidence
1	Strong evidence from at least one systematic review of multiple well-designed randomised, controlled trials
2	Strong evidence from at least one properly designed randomised, controlled trial of appropriate size
3	Evidence from well-designed trials without randomisation, single group pre-post, cohort, time series, or matched case-control studies
4	Evidence from well-designed non-experimental studies from more than one centre or research group
5	Opinions of respected authorities, based on clinical evidence, descriptive studies or reports of expert committees

From Muir-Gray (1997), copyright Elsevier.

Because of this and other compounding factors (such as perceptions and attitudes), there are high levels of health inequalities for this group of people. These factors, and the requirements within the Disability Discrimination Act (2005), dictate that additional measures, known as 'reasonable adjustments' must be taken to reduce the inequalities and remove barriers to access.

As the issue of general hospital care for people with a learning disability is a relatively new area of research (less than 20 years old), early studies provide good information to highlight the nature of the problem, but there are deficiencies in knowledge regarding interventions that may be effective in improving the process, and limited information is known about different stakeholder perspectives of the health care process.

Muir-Gray (1997, p. 61) describes five strengths of research evidence, which are illustrated in Table 1.2.

From this table it is apparent that the current evidence base is at Levels 4–5, with new research beginning to move this to Level 3. As this is a relatively new area of research that has only occurred within the past few years, knowledge is still developing, and further research is needed.

Dr. Mary Lindsay (1993) was one of the first professionals to identify access to health services for people with a learning disability as a problem area (Lindsay et al. 1993). In her original research, she found a literature search that revealed not a single article on the topic. She went on to chair the 1998 working party that produced *Signposts for Success* (NHSE 1998).

Signposts for Success explored the evidence base and highlighted:

a lack of good quality information on the effectiveness of many of the interventions used with people with learning disabilities and health related problems. The effectiveness of different models of health service delivery also requires further research. (NHSE 1998, p. 35)

They also state that:

It is unusual for research on general health problems to be specifically carried out on a learning disabled population. There are considerable ethical and methodological problems in carrying out randomised double blind controlled trials and these are a rarity. (NHSE 1998, p. 35)

This report further highlighted the issues and recommended that 'mainstream National Health Services (NHS) need to become more responsive to the special circumstances and needs of people with learning disabilities'. They also reported that people with learning disabilities 'have much higher needs than the general population yet visit the doctor less frequently, and use fewer preventative services. Services need to be more sensitive to their needs'.

Carers being required to provide basic care is a common finding in the evidence base along with:

- Illness or disease being missed or undiagnosed
- Poor understanding of specific health needs
- Negative attitudes of health care professionals
- Poor coordination of treatment
- Lack of accessible information
- Inappropriate use of control and restraint
- Inequality in service provision
- Need for training for health care professionals

Figure 1.2 illustrates the core themes relating to access to general hospital care, identified from the experiences of Acute Liaison Nurses (Learning Disability) in two trusts in England.

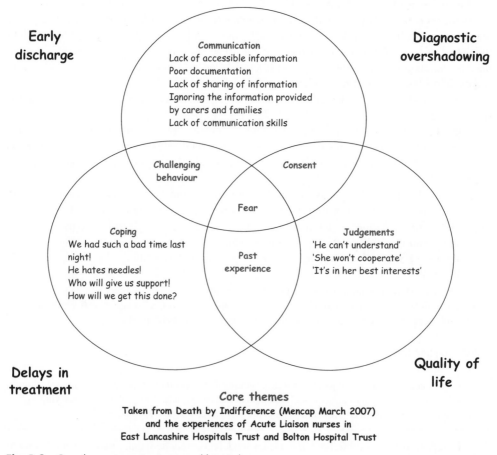

Early discharge

Diagnostic overshadowing

Communication
Lack of accessible information
Poor documentation
Lack of sharing of information
Ignoring the information provided
by carers and families
Lack of communication skills

Challenging behaviour

Consent

Fear

Coping
We had such a bad time last night!
He hates needles!
Who will give us support!
How will we get this done?

Past experience

Judgements
'He can't understand'
'She won't cooperate'
'It's in her best interests'

Delays in treatment

Quality of life

Core themes
Taken from Death by Indifference (Mencap March 2007)
and the experiences of Acute Liaison nurses in
East Lancashire Hospitals Trust and Bolton Hospital Trust

Fig. 1.2   Core themes in access to general hospital care.

Identifying and meeting the health needs of people with a learning disability

Over the past few centuries, much change in approach has occurred in the nature of caring for people with a learning disability. McClimens (cited in Grant et al. 2005, p. 31) reported that 'the care and treatment of individuals with a disability is traced to prehistoric times' and that 'medieval times saw the caring function performed by families, the Church or the local aristocracy'. The Poor Laws of 1601 show the beginnings of social policy seeking to address the needs of vulnerable people in society, leading to centuries of legislation and medical theory developing different models of care. McClimens (cited in Grant et al. 2005, p. 33) describes this as 'first a moral, then a legal and now a medical problem'.

The Human Rights Act (Department of Health 1998) highlighted that 'everyone has a right to expect and receive appropriate healthcare'. The UK Government clearly recognised an emerging area of need and commissioned a number of studies over the past few years relating to identifying and meeting the health needs of people with a learning disability. Mencap (2004) outlined the following key reasons why people with a learning disability have poorer health than the rest of the population:

1. *An increased risk of early death.* People with a learning disability are much more likely to die before the age of 50, and life expectancy is shortest for people who have the most support needs. The leading causes of death differ from those of the rest of the population. People with a learning disability:
   - Are three times more likely to die from respiratory disease
   - Have a higher risk of coronary heart disease (the second most common cause of death)
   - Have higher rates of gastrointestinal cancer and stomach disorders
2. *A higher prevalence of certain medical conditions.* It is known that people with a learning disability experience a greater variety, complexity and range of health problems than the rest of the population. This leads to a greater risk of poorer health and includes:
   - *Epilepsy*: 22% compared to 1% of the general population.
   - *Dementia*: 21.6% compared to 5.7% of the general population. People with Down's syndrome are also at a high risk of developing it younger.
   - *Schizophrenia*: 3% compared to 1% of the general population.
   - *Thyroid problems*: people with a learning disability, particularly those with Down's syndrome, have a greater risk of having thyroid problems.
   - *Osteoporosis*: tend to have osteoporosis younger than the general population and have more fractures.
   - *Sight problems*: more likely than the general population.
   - *Hearing problems*: 40% of people with a learning disability have hearing problems.
   - *Poor dental hygiene and dental care*: 36.5% of adults and 80% of adults with Down's syndrome have unhealthy teeth and gums.
   - *Underweight or overweight*: more likely to be under- or overweight than the general population.
   - *Mental health problems*: one in three people with a learning disability has problems with their mental health.
3. *Being part of a disadvantaged group in society.* People from disadvantaged groups have more illnesses and shorter lives than those who are well off. People with a learning disability are generally living on a low income. People with a learning disability from an ethnic minority are at an even greater disadvantage.

4. *Having unhealthy lifestyles.* People with a learning disability are often dependent on others to enable them to lead active lives. They are also dependent on others for what they eat. Less than 10% of adults with a learning disability eat a balanced diet, while 80% do less physical activity than is recommended.

The Royal College of Nursing (RCN) (2006) reported that 'the health of people with learning disabilities has steadily improved over the past 30 years; however, they still have higher levels of health needs than their non-learning disabled peers'. The RCN outline the following list of specific health needs of people with a learning disability, with further detail included in the publication of the rationale behind each of these needs:

- *Cancer*: different distribution from general population
- *Coronary heart disease*: the second highest cause of death
- *Dental issues/oral hygiene*
- *Diabetes*: higher than in the general population and may be attributed to increased levels of obesity, poor diet and inactive lifestyles
- *Epilepsy*: more prevalent and often more severe and complex than in the general population
- *Gastrointestinal problems*: including *Helicobacter pylori*, gastro-oesophageal reflux disease, constipation and coeliac disease
- *Mental health problems*: anxiety disorders, depression, schizophrenia
- Obesity: including links to some genetic conditions such as Prader–Willi syndrome
- *Respiratory disease*: the main cause of death in people with learning disabilities
- *Sensory impairments*: sight and hearing problems
- *Swallowing/feeding problems*: caused by neurological problems, structural abnormalities of the mouth, also rumination, regurgitation or self-induced vomiting
- *Thyroid disease/hypothyroidism*: annual blood tests for people with Down's syndrome are recommended

They also note that:

Although people with learning disabilities now live longer than they did decades ago they still have higher mortality rates than people without learning disabilities. People with more severe learning disabilities and people with Down's Syndrome have the shortest life expectancy. The highest causes of death for people with learning disabilities are respiratory disease followed by cardiovascular disease. The cardiovascular disease tends to be congenital rather than ischaemic. (RCN 2006)

The National Patient Safety Agency (NPSA) (2004) highlighted that their research confirmed that people with learning disabilities are more at risk of being involved in a patient safety incident than the general population. They identified a number of patient safety priorities as follows:

1. *Inappropriate use of physical intervention (control and restraint)* – people with learning disabilities may be receiving injuries and being harmed when physical restraint is used inappropriately. These should only be used when other less intrusive approaches have been tried and found to be ineffective.
2. *Vulnerability of people with a learning disability in hospitals* – more at risk of things going wrong than the general population, leading to varying degrees of harm being caused whilst in hospital.

3. *Swallowing difficulties (dysphagia)* – leading to respiratory tract infections, a leading cause of death for people with learning disabilities.
4. *Lack of accessible information* – people unable to understand information relating to illnesses, treatment or interventions.
5. *Illness or disease being mis- or undiagnosed* – leading to undetected health conditions and avoidable deaths.

Particular attention should be paid to feeding issues, and many people with a learning disability will need help to make their choice of food from menus. It is important to check if the person has any special dietary needs and how they usually take their food; does it need to be chopped up? What type of foods do they prefer and which utensils do they use? There may already be some specific feeding guidelines that their carers can pass on to you. A speech and language therapist should be consulted if there are any feeding or swallowing difficulties (e.g. choking and coughing). When feeding someone, you should attempt to make this a pleasant experience by sitting with the person, taking time with feeding and talking to them. Ensure meal is nicely presented, and they may wish to smell or touch the food, which should also be encouraged. Ensuring a person receives adequate nutrition and fluids is essential to their basic care during their stay in hospital, and a nominated individual should always take responsibility for monitoring this for people with a learning disability.

A person with Prader–Willi syndrome may have a tendency to overeat, and to eat inappropriate matter. You should seek specific advice from the Community Learning Disability Nurse about how to deal with eating/food issues for anyone with this syndrome.

Improved technology means that people with very complex and multiple health needs, who may not have done so previously, now survive and live longer. There are also improved interventions to support people to manage long-term complex health conditions. Both these reasons, in addition to the development of community-based care practices, mean that people with a learning disability and complex health needs are more likely to present in general hospitals than they did previously. Often health care professionals have limited contact with people with a learning disability, and it is an area where limited information is provided within their basic training. They often report a lack of knowledge and uncertainty when they have to care for someone with a learning disability.

Some learning disability conditions have associated specific health problems as a recognised feature of the condition, for example, the increased risk of developing hypothyroidism or Alzheimer's dementia in people with Down's syndrome, and regular health screening should be included as a routine process for people with these conditions. Whilst much of this is likely to take place with general practitioners in primary care services, it is also important for health care professionals in hospitals to develop an awareness of these specific health needs.

Learning disability varies a great deal between individuals, and what each individual needs to meet their health needs can also vary a great deal. Some people with a learning disability may find it difficult to adapt to a hospital environment, so the environment has to adapt more to them to accommodate and meet their needs (reasonable adjustments). Identifying how much and what kind of support each person needs is a key aspect of the health care process.

Mencap (1998) consulted widely with people with learning disabilities and their carers about their health care needs. They concluded:

> People with learning disabilities who stay in hospital for treatment often have to rely on carers to ensure their needs are met. This is because of a lack of pre-admission planning, lack of knowledge and confidence amongst staff about supporting someone with a learning disability, and inadequate staffing levels. (Mencap 1998)

Hart (1998) reported similar concern. Mencap (1998) highlighted a need for hospitals to 'have specific policies for people with learning disabilities, to ensure information exchange, and to meet the individual needs of people'. They believed that 'carers should not be expected to cover the care needs of a person with learning disabilities while they are a hospital inpatient'.

A number of strategies designed to increase the quality and effectiveness of general health care services were highlighted by Barr (1997), including pre-admission visits, assessment of needs, recognition of equal rights, coordinated teamwork, improved communication, and challenging stereotypes about people with learning disabilities. Each of these interventions needs further research to measure effectiveness and provide information for future service development.

The Health of the Nation for People with Learning Disabilities (Department of Health 1995a) recommended that 'people with learning disabilities should have access to all general health services ... with appropriate additional support as required to meet individual need'. The Mental Health Foundation (MHF) (1996), NHSE (1998) and Department of Health (1999) – all highlighted problems with access, understanding of health needs and appropriateness of services, with significant variation in practice across the country. Facing the Facts (Department of Health 1999) reported that health professionals were 'not in tune with the way that people with learning disabilities experience health interventions'.

The Department of Health commissioned the British Institute of Learning Disabilities to produce a report on secondary health care for people with learning disabilities. The authors, Cumella and Martin (2000), concluded that 'there is a broad consensus among service users, their families and professional carers, clinicians and managers about the kind of services needed to provide high quality secondary healthcare for people with learning disabilities'. They emphasise the need for a range of measures to improve communication, to support patients with a learning disability in hospital, and to improve the quality of health care.

Problems with access and poor understanding of health need were further highlighted in 'Valuing People' (Department of Health 2001a). The development of a health facilitator role is proposed as an intervention, and Bollard (2001) discusses how this role might be developed. Community Learning Disability Nurses are now recognised as a lead health care professional in acting in this health facilitator role. (*This role is explored further in Chapter 6.*)

Surprisingly, few professionals from hospital or learning disability services are familiar with the publication of the Royal College of Physicians (1998) Charter and Guidelines for Disabled People using Hospitals. The Charter, originally published in 1992, is based on the social model of disability, which identifies attitudes and the environment as being major causes of disability. It suggests that a named manager should be appointed in every hospital to deal with all disablement issues, and highlights a number of actions for hospitals to consider.

The Scottish NHSE (2002) published a national review of the contribution of nurses and midwives to the care and support of people with learning disabilities. They concluded that:

> As the largest group of care providers in NHS Scotland, nurses and midwives have a vital role in ensuring people with learning disabilities have their health needs met and gain access to services. *All* nurses and midwives – not just those who have chosen to specialise in caring for people with learning disabilities – need to work in partnership with people with learning disabilities and their family carers across health, social and education systems, in order to promote health and support inclusion. (Scottish NHSE 2002)

The Royal College of Nursing (2006) suggested some key approaches to meeting the health needs of people with a learning disability during an inpatient admission including:

- Assess needs before admission if possible
- Health care assistants to be aware of needs and to adapt practice as required
- A visit before admission can help, including meeting members of the team
- It is important for staff to 'engage' with the person and actively provide their care – some people may be very dependant on ward staff
- Use communication aids and show staff how to use them
- Use photographs
- Develop a routine/accessible timetable that includes ward round, mealtimes and other activities
- Flexible visiting hours
- Use written strategies for behavioural issues
- Incorporate activities that the person enjoys where possible
- Provide accessible information at discharge

Helping people with a learning disability get the best health treatment possible was the theme of the Mencap (2008) report 'Getting It Right'. The key message from this report is to 'see the person – not the disability', and the following are identified as important factors in meeting health needs:

✓ Find time to:
  - Listen to the person
  - Listen to the family
✓ Find the best way to communicate:
  - Pay attention to facial expressions
  - Notice gestures and body language
  - Try pointing to pictures
  - Try signing
✓ Keep information simple and brief
✓ Avoid using jargon

They continue to stress that it is important not to make assumptions about a person's quality of life and that people with a learning disability get ill and feel pain too. They recommend that health care professionals get to know some of the health conditions that are more common for people with a learning disability and that they act quickly ensuring they do not confuse a learning disability with illness.

In considering how the health needs of people with a learning disability can be met, HFT (2009) explain that 'the Government has responded in a number of ways, through legislation such as the Disability Discrimination Act (2005), and an Independent Inquiry into access to healthcare for people with learning disabilities, led by Sir Jonathon Michael'. The resulting report, Healthcare for All , highlighted that:

> High levels of health need are not currently being met and there are risks inherent in the care system. People with learning disabilities appear to receive less effective care than they are entitled to receive. There is evidence of a significant level of avoidable suffering and a high likelihood that there are deaths occurring which could be avoided (Michaels 2008, p. 53)

Whilst it was also acknowledged that there are examples of excellent practice in the process of health care, 'people with learning disabilities fare less well than other vulnerable groups in what can seem like a competition for political and local attention'.

The report made 10 principal recommendations about the 'reasonable adjustments' that are needed to make health care services as accessible to people with learning disabilities as they are to other people:

The Department of Health should:

1. Amend Core Standards for Better Health to include the requirement to make 'reasonable adjustments' to the provision and delivery of services.
2. Direct Primary Care Trusts to commission enhanced primary care services to include regular health checks for people with a learning disability.
3. Establish a learning disabilities public health observatory.

Trainers should:

4. Those with responsibility for the provision and regulation of undergraduate and postgraduate clinical training must ensure that curricula include mandatory training in learning disabilities.

Commissioners should:

5. Identify and assess the needs of people with learning disabilities and their carers, and use the information to inform the development of Local Area Agreements.

Providers should:

6. Ensure they collect data to identify people with a learning disability and track their pathways of care.
7. Trust boards should ensure they have effective systems in place to deliver 'reasonably adjusted' health services, including arrangements to provide advocacy for all those who need it.
8. Ensure the views and interests of people with learning disabilities and their carers are included in consultation for planning and development of services.
9. Involve family and carers as a matter of course as partners in the provision of treatment and care.

Inspectors and regulators should:

10. Develop and extend their monitoring of the standard of general health services provided for people with learning disabilities, in both the hospital sector and the community.

These recommendations, if fully implemented, provide a framework for identifying and meeting the health needs of people with a learning disability, with some being specific areas for general hospital services to consider. (*The ethical and political issues are explored further in Chapter 6.*)

Factors and barriers that influence the process of health care

As outlined earlier in this chapter, the current evidence base highlights that people with learning disabilities have increased health needs than the general population, yet their needs are often poorly understood, and sometimes not met. There is further evidence to suggest that some people experience difficulties in accessing appropriate health services to meet their needs (MHF 1996; NHSE 1998; Mencap 1998, 2004, 2008; Department of Health 1999, 2001a). Some of the key factors and barriers highlighted include:

- Hospital staff not understanding the specific health needs of people with learning disabilities.
- Problems with communication and behaviour.
- Under- or overprotectiveness.
- Carers having to stay with people to provide basic care.
- Negative attitudes and a lack of confidence of hospital staff working with people with learning disabilities.

The Royal College of Nursing (2006, p. 4) highlighted a number of other factors that influence why people with learning disabilities might not access the health services they need including:

- The philosophy of care in learning disability services moving from a medical to a social model.
- Confusion about consent leading to delays in treatment.
- Health screening not offered if people are not considered to be at risk (e.g. cervical screening).
- Barriers to attending such as poor physical access to health services and the expense of travelling to appointments.
- The need for support to access services.
- Signs and symptoms being attributed to the learning disability condition, rather than other causes, including ill health (known as *diagnostic overshadowing*).
- Health problems might be accompanied by unusual signs and symptoms.
- Health promotion materials may not be accessible to people with learning disabilities.
- People might have difficulties communicating and may not be aware of the health services available to them.
- People might be less inclined to take up screening if they do not understand the benefits.
- People may not understand the consequences their decisions can have on their health needs.

A number of other key factors that contribute to discriminatory practice which can influence the process of health care were identified by Mencap (2007) including:

1. People with a learning disability are seen to be a low priority.
2. Many health care professionals do not understand much about learning disability.
3. Many health care professionals do not properly consult and involve the families and carers of people with a learning disability.
4. Many health care professionals do not understand the law around capacity and consent to treatment.
5. Health professionals rely inappropriately on their estimates of a person's quality of life.
6. The complaint system within NHS services is often ineffectual, time-consuming and inaccessible.

Whilst all these factors may present challenges to health care professionals, there is evidence of positive experiences. Mencap (2004) consulted with 1000 people with a learning disability and showed high levels of satisfaction with the health services received, but they did also show examples of poor experiences.

Hannon (2003) undertook a research project which included exploring the experiences of people with a learning disability admitted to hospital for treatment. The results from this study show a much more positive experience than expected for people with a learning disability involved in a hospital admission. Whilst this was only a relatively small sample size, a good evaluation of health care was received, with good correlation of feedback across all stakeholder groups. Some of the key factors that influenced the health care process included:

- The nursing process – assess, plan, implement and evaluate – provided the basis for care planning in this project. All admissions were seen as successful in terms of treatment being completed. Everyone welcomed short admissions.
- The levels of support needed for people with a learning disability in hospital vary widely, and need to be assessed for each individual. Some people require little additional support, whilst others may need one-to-one support throughout their stay. Time is important, for physical and emotional support, and time to be with the person. Each individual needs a person-centred care plan that is flexible and responsive to their individual needs.
- Carers provide various levels of support, from occasional visits to 24-hour care. Carers generally felt this was for the service user's benefit. They felt that learning disability nurses are better able to communicate with hospital staff than they are, and also that hospital staff are more likely to listen to another professional.
- Very little environmental change is needed. Most people are able to mix with other patients, and blend into usual ward surroundings and activities. Whilst the choice of a single room is appropriate for some people, there is no need to put people there as a matter of course. This continues to isolate people within secondary health care services, and within the wider community.
- Hospital staff are more confident with more able people, but less so where there are any behaviour or communication problems, or other complex needs. They find it difficult to judge levels of functioning when people present as being more able than they actually are. A difference in approach is evident with hospital staff who had spent time in learning disability services. The experienced hospital staff in this study perhaps contributed to successful admissions.
- Of the key problems highlighted in the evidence base, the lack of knowledge, lack of confidence and negative attitudes did not seem to reflect the personal qualities of the staff, but rather a lack of experience, training and preparation to work with people with a learning disability. All hospital staff in this study showed a caring response and a willingness to learn. They felt they had a lack of information about learning disability, what it is and what it means for the individual, and that this should be included within their basic nurse training.

(See also section on pre-admission in Chapter 2.)

Considering feedback from the key stakeholders within this project, hospital staff valued carers staying with the person but mainly saw this as being of benefit to the service user rather than themselves. Many hospital staff were not aware that the majority of people with a learning disability live at home with their families. Hospital staff gave the highest overall rating scores (evaluating aspects of hospital admission) of all stakeholder groups. Whilst this is based on what they perceived as positive outcomes, this perhaps also reflects a sense of relief that the admission had been better than they expected. They were pleased that no problems were highlighted, they felt prepared and supported, and all admissions were successful in terms of completing treatment. The fact that hospital staff rated the stay of a person with a learning disability on their ward as 'excellent' also indicates a more positive attitude than was expected, and they may have responded differently before taking part in the study.

Hospital staff had a positive attitude towards learning disability nurses even though knew little about them, and the training they completed. They were complimentary about the input of learning disability nurses, appreciated their support, and thought their intervention was very effective. The interventions from learning disability nurses closely correlated with strategies suggested by Barr (1997), designed to increase the quality and effectiveness of general health care services. They also supported the results reported by Davis and Marsden (2001).

The following are examples of factors that influenced the health care process during a hospital admission – reported from a focus group also undertaken as part of this project:

- The hospital admission was generally a positive experience, better than expected in comparison with evidence base.
- One bad experience involving another patient calling a person with a learning disability names was very distressing for the person involved.
- Service users showed a good understanding of their health needs, reason for admission and treatment received.
- People felt they were treated the same as everyone else, and had a positive attitude towards hospital staff.
- Support for carers is important.
- It is good to be prepared and take things with you that you need.
- Communication can be a problem. Suggested hospital staff use Makaton symbols and pictures. (*See Chapter 3 for information about Makaton.*)
- Things that help include being told what is going to happen, people explaining things, asking people what is wrong with them, and having support for the person.

One of the other key areas for consideration is the issue of patient safety. The National Patient Safety Agency (2004) in its document 'Listening to People with Learning Difficulties and Family Carers Talk About Patient Safety' highlighted a number of issues relating to the safety of people with learning disabilities accessing primary and secondary health care. The 12 most commonly talked about areas of concern for the people consulted were:

1. Lack of contact with primary health care services
2. Prescribing medication
3. The need for information in accessible formats
4. Treating depression
5. Care for people with severe mental health problems
6. Practical support when in hospital
7. Anxiety about being in hospital
8. The effect of long waiting times
9. Communication between health and social care services
10. Services for people with high support needs
11. Health awareness and screening
12. Informing health services when things go wrong

Whilst a number of these areas are related to primary care services, the majority are also relevant for health care professionals in general hospitals. (*See relevant sections in each chapter for more information regarding these issues.*)

Reflective Learning Point:

What patient safety concerns would you have about a person with a learning disability accessing the area you work in?

Many of the people consulted by NPSA talked about finding being admitted to hospital stressful and frightening. This may lead to people with learning disabilities avoiding having procedures and discharging themselves early. Some people felt lonely being in hospital and wanted more attention from staff. It was noted that those people who received attention felt it had a positive effect.

For some people the anxiety is related to not being informed about what is happening. It is important to acknowledge that not everyone will understand what it means to have their blood pressure taken or have an x-ray. Being fully informed about treatment is important in preventing undue stress and anxiety. Another important issue to consider is that some people with learning disabilities may have memories of living in long-stay hospitals and the experience of institutional living. This may result in the person feeling fearful of not being discharged home or of experiencing aspects of institutional care that they did not like.

Overcoming barriers to care

People with a learning disability represent a wide and diverse range of conditions and associated health problems, and their actual reason for hospital admission may be completely unrelated to their disability. As explored earlier in this chapter, the perception and attitude of the health care professional can create a barrier before they even meet the person. The following summarises the key difficulties and barriers that influence the health care process:

- Hospital staff not understanding the specific health needs of people with learning disabilities.
- Problems with communication and behaviour.
- Under- or overprotectiveness.
- Carers having to stay with people to provide basic care.
- Negative attitudes and a lack of confidence of hospital staff working with people with learning disabilities.
- Confusion about consent leading to delays in treatment.
- Health screening not offered if people are not considered to be at risk (e.g. cervical screening).
- Barriers to attending such as poor physical access to health services and the expense of travelling to appointments.
- The need for support to access services.
- Signs and symptoms being attributed to the learning disability condition, rather than other causes, including ill health (known as *diagnostic overshadowing*).
- Health problems might be accompanied by unusual signs and symptoms.
- Health promotion materials may not be accessible to people with learning disabilities.

- People might have difficulties communicating and may not be aware of the health services available to them.
- People might be less inclined to take up screening if they do not understand the benefits.
- People may not understand the consequences their decisions can have on their health needs.

Whilst these factors and barriers may present challenges to health care professionals, it can sometimes be just simple adaptations to the usual process of care that can make the experience more comfortable for all concerned. These are suggestions of adaptations that could be helpful:

- Avoid long waiting periods and allow extra time for tasks.
- Having a cubicle that has as little equipment as possible on view.
- Taking a mobile telephone number so that the patient and carer can leave the waiting area until it is time to be seen.
- Being creative in producing health promotion resources.
- Minimising the number of people having to assess and treat the patient.
- Identify tests that can be carried out at the same time (especially if sedation is being used) to minimise distress for the person.
- Speaking to the carer away from the patient (if the patient lacks capacity and it is agreed that it is in the patient's best interest to prevent distress to talk away from the patient).
- Remember to talk to the person, especially to explain what is happening during health interventions, but also just to pass the time of day.
- Utilise the skills of other professionals in the unit. Hospital play coordinators may have some useful distraction activities or equipment that may be appropriate.

It is of no surprise that waiting time is a common concern for people with learning disabilities and their family or carers, especially those with complex needs. The time spent waiting often causes the person to become anxious, and therefore their ability to focus on the consultation and answer questions or be able to tolerate tests or investigations is very much affected. Making the appointment at the start of the list is an obvious solution to ensure that the person is seen as near to the appointment time as possible. It is also important for the health care professional leading the clinic to be aware of any problems occurring in the waiting area and to respond as quickly as possible when the patient needs to be seen as soon as possible, which may require them being seen before another patient. From experience of sitting with an anxious patient, other patients waiting are very supportive and are more concerned for the person's anxiety than missing their turn.

Reflective Learning Point:

Think about a situation where you have had to make 'reasonable adjustments' to overcome a barrier and enable health care to be provided to someone. How did this make you feel?

Hannon (2003) reported feedback from a focus group of people with learning disabilities who had been in hospital who suggested:

Things that help (with health interventions) include; being told what is going to happen, people explaining things, asking the person what is wrong with them, and support for the person. Some people need more help than others, and carers need support to provide shared care.

One of the significant factors the group identified was time – time for explanation and time to be with the person. This could create resource problems when someone is admitted needing a high level of support. It was useful to do an introductory visit for some people, meet staff and be shown around. This was seen as part of the 'health facilitator' role of the Community Learning Disability Nurse (*see further information in Chapter 6*). They also felt it is important to be involved in discharge planning, and thought this did not often happen because of a lack of awareness of their role.

Community Learning Disability Nurses particularly highlighted communication and behaviour needs. They made the point that some people with a learning disability may present as being more capable than they actually are, and hospital staff do not always pick this up. (*See earlier notes on how to establish if your patient has a learning disability*.) Hospital staff need to 'positively discriminate' with regards to providing the health care needed to meet the person's needs.

FAMILY/CARER'S NEEDS

People with complex health conditions now live longer, and the demand for care will continue to grow. Caring for a person with a learning disability can often be considered to be a lifelong role. The Department of Health (2008) strategy gave the following definition of a carer: 'A carer spends a significant proportion of their life providing unpaid support to family or potentially friends. This could be caring for a relative, partner or friend who is ill, frail, disabled or has mental health or substance misuse problems'.

Reflective Learning Point:

Write a list of what you think would be the main needs of a carer of a person with a learning disability and how these could best be met.

Michael (2008, p. 20) in his report 'Healthcare for All' highlighted that:

One in 8 people (around 5.2 million altogether in England and Wales) is a carer. Most carers (58%) are women and some are children. Around 60% of carers look after someone with a disability, 15% care for someone with mental and physical ill health and/or a learning disability, and 7% care for someone with a mental health problem alone.

The inquiry team that produced this report held two consultation meetings with family members and carers of people with a learning disability. The most common concerns highlighted by carers related to the quality of care during a hospital admission for people with learning disabilities. The following key points were highlighted in their feedback (see Annex 5 in report) (cited in Michael 2008):

- Attitudes and values of health care professionals and the effect on health care provided.
- Gaps in communication, and problems with finding a balance between communicating with the person with a learning disability and the carer. Some staff did not communicate with the carer at all.
- The importance of clear accessible information.
- Gaps in partnership working, for example between primary and secondary care.

- Consideration of carers' needs, such as:
  - Taking account of their knowledge of the person with a learning disability.
  - Services working together with carers.
  - Services not being too dependent on carers to provide care, yet should provide carers with support to stay with the person if needed.
  - Carers often also have responsibility for other family members.
  - Carers may have their own unmet physical health care needs.

In the Michael (2008, p. 20) report, one carer (mother) explained:

> My daughter needs 24/7 care and when she is in hospital I or another person who knows her well have to stay with her . . . I often have to sleep in her wheelchair, or the seat by her bed, or a mattress on the floor if I am lucky. I am not offered a drink or food, or access to a toilet for myself.

It is important for health care professionals to consider 'Who is the carer?' For people with a learning disability, this could be a family member/relatives, paid or unpaid carers, health or social care professionals – who may be qualified or not. The carer, particularly if a family member, may have many years of experience in caring for the individual. It is important for health care professionals to develop a relationship with the carers at an early stage in the health care process. They have much knowledge to share about the person, and listening to them now will prove to be valuable later.

It is vital to exchange information with the carers as they need to have a full understanding of the reason for admission, and any health interventions or procedures required. All carers will provide a valuable source of information, advice, guidance and support when caring for someone with a learning disability, and the importance of their contribution towards a successful hospital stay cannot be underestimated. Health care professionals must be prepared to listen to the carers and accept their advice about the best way of dealing with the individual they are caring for.

Mencap (1998) consulted with people with learning disabilities and their carers and concluded that people with a learning disability admitted to hospital often rely on the carers to provide basic care for the individual during their hospital stay. Whilst carers are usually happy to offer both their physical and emotional support to the individual, sometimes carers are expected to do too much and provide basic care that should be provided by the hospital team. This is not acceptable practice and health care professionals should not expect carers to undertake caring duties. It is the responsibility of the hospital to provide whatever care the person needs, including making any reasonable adjustments necessary to meet these needs.

Health care professionals need to be aware that the carer also has needs, and it is important to care for the carers and identify and meet their needs too. It should be remembered that the carer may themselves be anxious and emotional about the visit to hospital, and that they may transfer their own anxiety onto the individual, and need reassurance themselves. This may be a combination of anxiety about the health and well-being of the individual, but may also include their own concerns about dealing with health care professionals and feeling confused in the hospital environment. In order for them to offer the best support to the individual and the health care professionals caring for them, it is important they know what the health condition is and that they actually understand themselves what is going on. They may feel a lack of control about what is happening to the person, and it is important they are kept fully informed. Carers are often unsure about how much is expected of them, and they may also have other caring responsibilities that they need to continue. Helping carers to manage their anxiety will help to support the person during their hospital stay and contribute to successful interventions.

Hannon (2003) reported that carers who stayed with individuals in hospital were happy with the support they received from hospital staff, and were positive about the multidisciplinary teamwork. They felt hospital staff do not always understand people with a learning disability, although this improves as they get to know the person. Carers worried about other patients being disturbed and felt it is acceptable, when appropriate, to put people in single rooms. They felt it is important to have familiar people around, and appreciated support from the learning disability nurse.

The Department of Health (2008) strategy for carers recognises the important role that carers play and acknowledges that carers need more help and support than has been available in the past. In this report carers explained (Department of Health 2008, p. 1, of summary report) that they want 'a system that helps them to manage the twin demands of work and caring responsibilities'. They want 'more personalised support and greater scope to control and customise services, including in healthcare where identifying needs and prompt access to services can be so critical'.

The report summarised (Department of Health 2008, p. 62) the largest categories for comments from 79 carers during the public consultation as follows:

- The importance of listening to carers (58% mentioned this)
- The need for better education and training for staff (55%)
- The problem of communication (52%)
- Better information and signposting (22%)
- The importance of being flexible about appointments and taking sufficient time (32%)
- Shortage of resources (32%)
- The importance of being able to stay close to their relative when in hospital (25%)
- The value of liaison or link workers (31%)

The 10-year strategy outlines a vision to be achieved by 2018 for carers to be respected as 'expert care partners', with access to the services they need to support them in their caring role. Specific mention was made of carers' relationship with the NHS: 'Carers have called for closer working between the NHS, Social Services and themselves'. To encourage this, pilot sites have been established to examine how the NHS can better support carers and this will involve:

- The active involvement of carers in diagnosis, care and discharge planning
- Greater support for carers at GP practices and hospitals
- Closer working with councils and voluntary organisations

They also highlight a need to pay attention to the health and well-being of carers, including introducing pilots of annual health checks for carers, and improving emotional support for carers.

INTRODUCTION TO PERSON-CENTRED APPROACHES

Person-centred approaches are very familiar to anyone working within learning disability practice. O Brian and Lovett (1992) set the agenda for a new model of working with people with learning disabilities. They defined person-centred planning as:

Refers to a family of approaches to organising and guiding community change in alliance with people with disabilities and their families and friends. Person-centred planning approaches include: Individual Service Design, Essential Lifestyle Planning, Personal Futures Planning, MAPS (Making Action Plans) and PATH (Planning Alternative Tomorrows with Hope). (O Brian and Lovett 1992)

Each of these approaches includes a range of techniques designed to enable a person-centred plan to be developed. Any or all of these approaches may be in use with a person with a learning disability, and their family/carer should be asked to explain about the person's plan if there is one in place. Your local Learning Disability Nurses can explain about the conceptual and theoretical framework, and provide examples of what a plan may look like.

The Department of Health (2001b) defines 'person-centred planning' as:

A process for continual listening and learning, focusing on what is important to someone now and in the future, and acting upon this in alliance with their family and friends. This listening is used to understand a person's capacities and choices. Person-centred planning is the basis for problem solving and negotiation to mobilise the necessary resources to pursue a person's aspirations.

This theme is continued in the white paper 'Valuing People' (Department of Health 2001a), with the requirement to develop person-centred individual Health Action Plans for people with a learning disability. Valuing People (Department of Health 2001a) defined the key aspects of person-centred planning as:

- The person being at the centre of the process
- Listening to and learning from what people want from their lives
- Helping people to think about what they want now and in the future
- Family and friends working together with the person to make this happen
- Reflecting the person's capabilities and specifying the level of support required

It is important to note that this approach applies to all areas of the individuals' life and not just to their time spent in hospital. Some people may present with a plan that has been specifically written for their hospital stay, and for others it may be an overall plan for how they access the health care services they need as part of maintaining a healthy lifestyle.

Person-centred approaches are based on the principles of humanistic psychology, and are about enabling the transfer of control and personal empowerment to the client from the person working with them. Carl Rogers is regarded as the founder, in the 1940s, of the person-centred approach. This was originally called 'client-centred therapy' as opposed to 'patient-centred', reflecting Rogers' belief that people, not therapists, know what is best for themselves. Jukes and Aldridge (2006, p. 1) explain that 'the premise is that the person is of centrality in the professional relationship, and that effective person-centred practices are based around skilled interactional and interpersonal processes'. They continue to state (Jukes and Aldridge 2006, p. 10) that, with regard to health care, what patients want is care which:

1. Explores the patient's main reason for the visit, concerns and need for information
2. Seeks an integrated understanding of the patient's world – that is, their whole person, emotional needs and life issues
3. Finds common ground on what the problem is and mutually agrees on management
4. Enhances prevention and health promotion
5. Enhances the continuing relationship between the patient and the health care professional

Table 1.3   The seven Pendleton 'tasks'

1. Define the reason for the patient's attendance (ideas, concerns and expectations)
2. Consider other problems (continuing and 'at risk' areas)
3. Work with the patient to choose an appropriate action for each problem
4. Achieve a shared understanding of the problem
5. Involve the patient in the management and encourage the acceptance of responsibility
6. Use time and resources appropriately
7. Establish a relationship, which helps to achieve other tasks

From Pendleton et al. (1984). By permission of Oxford University Press.

The concept of patient-centred approaches became more visible in the 1980s when Pendleton et al. (1984) (cited in Jukes and Aldridge 2006, p. 9) suggested that good practice should be based on what is known as the Pendleton 'tasks', illustrated in Table 1.3.

These principles form the basis of how health care professionals work with patients, with the emphasis on developing a 'helping relationship'. Jukes and Aldridge (2006, p. 13) continue to explain that:

> Person-centredness does offer different definitions and applications within different care arenas. They do, however, have a common thread which represents a cohesive approach. The person/patient is at the heart of practice and communication along with an attitude of value, equality, respect and partnership in care between the professional and patient/client. The ability to listen, engage and form an alliance is its central tenet.

Using person-centred approaches enables the health care professional to see the person with a learning disability as a valued individual with the equal right to receive the health care they need.

Whilst the concept of person-centred approaches may not yet be as familiar in general hospital services, it is beginning to influence clinical practice. Binnie and Titchen (1999) describe a project that successfully transformed a traditional task-based care delivery system within a hospital medical unit into a patient-centred service. They suggest (Binnie & Titchen 1999, p. 234) that 'developing patient centred practice means being prepared to review, and possibly to change, virtually every aspect of ward life'. The importance of the role of the 'leader' in influencing and facilitating this change in practice is demonstrated throughout the book and they explain (Binnie & Titchen 1999, p. 234) that 'experiential learning in a ward is facilitated by the presence of a senior practitioner who can demonstrate the living reality of patient-centred nursing and who can help nurses to learn from what they see, what they do and what they feel in their everyday work'. This closely correlates with the evidence base outlined earlier in this chapter, where it was clear that working with an experienced and confident practitioner when caring for a person with a learning disability really makes a difference.

Person-centred care is about being flexible and responsive to individual needs, and health care professionals who work within this philosophy will develop a more therapeutic relationship with the person and you will approach the way you work with them differently. Binnie and Titchen (1999, p. 171) reported numerous scenarios that were part of their research project and found that 'the nurses ability to "be with" their patients seemed greatly to enhance their ability to work with them'. Campbell (1984) described this as 'being with and not just doing to'. The patient's status changes from passive recipient of health care to that of an active partner engaged in the health care process. There may be significant barriers to overcome in order to practice this when working with people with a learning disability, but the rewards will feel worth it. (*See more on developing relationships in Chapter 3.*)

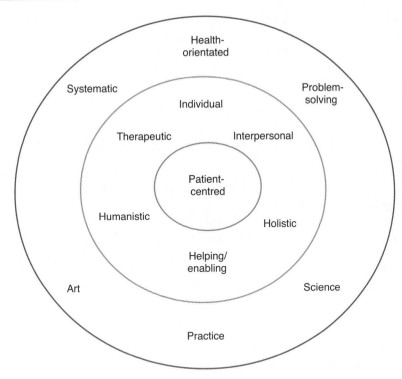

Fig. 1.3 Key attributes of nursing. Savage (2007) cited in RCN (2007). Reproduced with the kind permission of the RCN.

Figure 1.3 illustrates the key attributes of nursing using a person-centred approach – identified by Savage (1998) reported in RCN (2007).

Hannon (2003) found that although person-centred approaches were not familiar to hospital staff in her study, they found they could be effectively developed and implemented in secondary health care services. Hospital staff showed positive regard for service users and spent time helping people to settle. There was evidence of person-centred approaches being used, and services were responsive to individual needs. They were flexible and maintained usual routines for people where possible. One hospital staff felt going into hospital can be 'scary for a healthy person', and this could be aggravated by having a learning disability. Hospital staff also made comparisons with other vulnerable groups – elderly, confused, people with physical disabilities, people who could not read or write, or had poor eyesight – and felt that detailed pre-admission planning based on person-centred approaches, as implemented in this study, would be beneficial for the other vulnerable groups too. (*See further information on pre-admission assessment in Chapter 2.*)

CONCLUSION

This chapter sets out to provide an introduction to the nature of learning disability and insight into what this means for the person. A diagnosis of a learning disability has a lifelong impact on the person and their family/carers. Health care professionals need to develop a greater awareness and understanding of how to identify and meet the health needs of people with a learning disability. Working with experienced and confident people can help, and listening to and working with families/carers can support health care professionals to provide the best care possible. Person-centred approaches enable individual care plans to be developed that are flexible and responsive to individual needs.

Summary of Key Learning Points

The key learning points are:
- It is important to establish the presence of a learning disability early in the health care process.
- A diagnosis of a learning disability can help you to identify specific health needs that may be associated with this, which are more prevalent in people with a learning disability than in the general population.
- The perception and attitude of health care professionals influence the care you provide to people with a learning disability and can create a barrier to effective health care.
- People with a learning disability have a wide range of complex health needs, with some specific health conditions being more prevalent in this group than in the general population.
- Health services are required to make 'reasonable adjustments' to enable people with a learning disability to access the health care they need.
- It is important to work in partnership with carers and also remember to consider their needs.
- Person-centred approaches that are flexible and responsive to individual needs provide a framework for working with people with a learning disability to identify and meet their health needs.

Links to KSF Competencies – Chapter 1

| | Level descriptors | | | |
	1	2	3	4
Core dimensions				
1 – Communication	Communicate with a limited range of people on day-to-day matters	Communicate with a range of people on a range of matters	Develop and maintain communication with people about difficult matters and/or in difficult situations	Develop and maintain communication with people on complex matters, issues and ideas and/or in complex situations
2 – Personal and people development	Contribute to own personal development	Develop own skills and knowledge and provide information to others to help their development	Develop oneself and contribute to the development of others	Develop oneself and others in areas of practice
3 – Health safety and security	Assist in maintaining own and others' health, safety and security	Monitor and maintain health, safety and security of self and others	Promote, monitor and maintain the best practice in health, safety and security	Maintain and develop an environment and culture that improves health, safety and security

4 – Service improvement	Make changes in own practice and offer suggestions for improving services	Contribute to the improvement of services	Appraise, interpret and apply suggestions, recommendations and directives to improve services	Work in partnership with others to develop, take forward and evaluate direction, policies and strategies
5 – Quality	Maintain the quality of own work	Maintain quality in own work and encourage others to do so	Contribute to improving quality	Develop a culture that improves quality
6 – Equality and diversity	Act in ways that support equality and value diversity	Support equality and value diversity	Promote equality and value diversity	Develop a culture that promotes equality and value diversity
Health and well-being				
HWB1 – Promotion of health and well-being and prevention of adverse effects on health and well-being	Contribute to promoting health and well-being and preventing adverse effects on health and well-being	Plan, develop and implement approaches to promote health and well-being and prevent adverse effects on health and well-being	Plan, develop and implement programmes to promote health and well-being and prevent adverse effects on health and well-being	Promote health and well-being and prevent adverse effects on health and well-being through contributing to the development, implementation and evaluation of related policies
HWB2 – Assessment and care planning to meet health and well-being needs	Assist in the assessment of people's health and well-being needs	Contribute to assessing health and well-being needs and planning how to meet those needs	Assess health and well-being needs and develop, monitor and review care plans to meet specific needs	Assess complex health and well-being needs and develop, monitor and review care plans to meet those needs
HWB3 – Protection of health and well-being	Recognise and report situations where there might be a need for protection	Contribute to protecting people at risk	Implement aspects of a protection plan and review its effectiveness	Develop and lead on the implementation of an overall protection plan
HWB4 – Enablement to address health and well-being needs	Help people meet daily health and well-being needs	Enable people to meet ongoing health and well-being needs	Enable people to address specific needs in relation to health and well-being	Empower people to realise and maintain their potential in relation to health and well-being
HWB5 – Provision of care to meet health and well-being needs	Undertake care activities to meet individuals' health and well-being needs	Undertake care activities to meet the health and well-being needs of individuals, with a greater degree of dependency	Plan, deliver and evaluate care to meet people's health and well-being needs	Plan, deliver and evaluate care to address people's complex health and well-being needs

HWB6 – Assessment and treatment planning	Undertake tasks related to the assessment of physiological and psychological functioning	Contribute to the assessment of physiological and psychological functioning	Assess physiological and psychological functioning and develop, monitor and review related treatment plans	Assess physiological and psychological functioning when there are complex and/or undifferentiated abnormalities, diseases and disorders and develop, monitor and review related treatment plans
HWB7 – Interventions and treatments	Assist in providing interventions and/or treatments	Contribute to planning, delivering and monitoring interventions and/or treatments	Plan, deliver and evaluate interventions and/or treatments	Plan, deliver and evaluate interventions and/or treatments when there are complex issues and/or serious illness

Department of Health (2004). Reproduced under the terms of the Click-Use Licence.

REFERENCES

Barr O (1997) Care of people with learning disabilities in hospital. *Nursing Standard*, 12(8), 49–56.

Biley A M (1994) A handicap of negative attitudes and lack of choice: caring for inpatients with disabilities. *Professional Nurse*, 9(12), 786–788.

Binnie A and Titchen A (1999) *Freedom to Practice: The Development of Patient-centred Nursing*. Butterworth Heinemann, Oxford.

Bollard M (2001) New roles, new opportunities. *Learning Disability Practice*, 4(4), 10–12.

British Psychological Society (2000) *Learning Disability: Definitions and Contexts*. BSP, Leicester.

Campbell A V (1984) *Moderated Love: A Theology of Professional Care*. SPCK, London.

Cumella S and Martin D (2000) *Secondary Healthcare for People with a Learning Disability*. BILD, Birmingham.

Davis S and Marsden R (2001) Disabled people in hospital: evaluating the Clinical Nurse Specialist (CNS) role. *Nursing Standard*, 15(21), 33–37.

Department of Health (1983) *The Mental Health Act*. HMSO, London.

Department of Health (1995a) *The Health of the Nation for People with Learning Disabilities*. HMSO, London.

Department of Health (1995b) *Disability Discrimination Act*. HMSO, London.

Department of Health (1998) *Human Rights Act*. HMSO, London.

Department of Health (1999) *Facing the Facts*. HMSO, London.

Department of Health (2001a) *Valuing People*. HMSO, London.

Department of Health (2001b) *Planning with People: Towards Person-Centred Approaches – Guidance for Implementation Groups*. HMSO, London.

Department of Health (2004) *The NHS Knowledge and Skills Framework (NHS KSF) and the Development Review Process. Appendix 1: Overview of the NHS KSF*. HMSO, London.

Department of Health (2008) *Carers at the Heart of 21st Century Families and Communities: A Caring System on Your Side, a Life of Your Own*. HMSO, London.

Disability Discrimination Act (2005) The Stationery Office: London.

Emerson E and Hatton C (2004) *Estimating the Current Need/Demand for Support for People with Learning Disabilities in England*. Lancaster University, UK.

Fitzsimmons J and Barr O (1997) A review of the reported attitudes of health and social care professionals towards people with learning disabilities: implications for education and further research. *Journal of Learning Disabilities for Nursing, Health and Social Care*, 1(2), 57–64.

Grant G, Goward P, Richardson M and Ramcharan P (2005) *Learning Disability – A Life Cycle Approach to Valuing People*. Open University Press, Maidenhead.

Hannon L (2003) *Pre-admission Assessment in Secondary Healthcare Services for People with Learning Disabilities*. Unpublished MSc Dissertation. University of Central Lancashire, UK.

Hart S (1998) Learning-disabled people's experience of general hospitals. *British Journal of Nursing*, 7(8), 470–477.

HFT (2009) *Working Together: Easy Steps to Improving How People with a Learning Disability are Supported When in Hospital (Guidance for Hospitals, Families and Paid Support Staff)*. HFT, Gloucester, UK.

Jukes M and Aldridge J (2006) *Person-Centred Practices: A Therapeutic Perspective*. Quay, London.

Lindsay M, Singh K and Perrett A (1993) Management of learning disability in the general hospital. *British Journal of Hospital Medicine*, 50, 182–186.

Mencap (1998) *Health for All*. Mencap, London.

Mencap (2002) *'Quality of Life' and Medical Decision Making for Adults with Profound and Multiple Learning Disabilities*. Mencap, London.

Mencap (2004) *Treat Me Right! Better Healthcare for People with a Learning Disability*. Mencap, London.

Mencap (2007) *Death by Indifference*. Mencap, London.

Mencap (2008) *Getting It Right When Treating People with a Learning Disability*. Mencap, London.

Mental Health Foundation (MHF) (1996) *Building Expectations*. MHF, London.

Michaels J (2008) *Healthcare for All. Report of the Independent Inquiry into Access to Healthcare for People with Learning Disabilities*. HMSO, London.

Muir-Gray J A (1997) *Evidence-Based Healthcare. How to Make Health Policy and Management Decisions*. Churchill Livingstone, Glasgow.

National Patient Safety Agency (NPSA) (2004) *Listening to People with Learning Difficulties and Family Carers Talk About Patient Safety*. NPSA, London.

NHS Executive (1998) *Signposts for Success*. HMSO, London.

O Brian J and Lovett H (1992) *Finding a Way Towards Everyday Lives: The Contribution of Person Centred Planning*. Pennsylvania Office of Mental Retardation, Harrisburg.

Pendleton D, Schofield T, Tate P and Havelock P (1984) *The Consultation: An Approach to Learning and Teaching*. Oxford University Press, Oxford.

Royal College of Nursing (2006) *Meeting the Health Needs of People with Learning Disabilities: Guidance for Nursing Staff*. RCN, London.

Royal College of Nursing (2007) *Defining Nursing*. RCN, London.

Royal College of Physicians (1998) *Disabled People Using Hospitals: A Charter and Guidelines*. RCP, London.

Scottish NHS Executive (2002) *Promoting Health, Supporting Inclusion*. NHSE, Edinburgh.

Shanley E and Guest C (1995) Stigmatisation of people with learning disabilities in general hospitals. *British Journal of Nursing*, 4(13), 759–760.

Slevin E and Sines D (1996) Attitudes of nurses in a general hospital towards people with learning disabilities: influence of contact, and graduate/non-graduate status, a comparative study. *Journal of Advanced Nursing*, 24, 1116–1126.

2 The Process of Health Care

INTRODUCTION

This chapter focuses on the process of health care and the patient journey from admission to discharge through different areas of a general hospital. It includes a particular focus on the pre-admission part of the process and introduces a number of care pathways to support health care professionals with care planning. The overall aim is to provide health care professionals with best practice guidance on how to provide health interventions to people with a learning disability, including advice on the practical support that is needed. The chapter concludes by highlighting the key points to consider when discharge planning.

Going into hospital for any reason can cause anxiety, worry and confusion for anyone. The HFT guidance 'Working Together' (2009) highlights that 'People are often unsure of what to expect or how they will cope' and that for someone who has a learning disability, this experience is likely to be even more complicated for a wide range of reasons: 'They are likely to find it more difficult to communicate natural anxieties or explain any pain or discomfort they may be in. They may have difficulty in adjusting to the hospital environment and routines. The hospital staff may not know or understand their cognitive, health and personal care needs. They may also have had poor experiences of health care in the past. Such vulnerability is likely to be further increased by other factors like epilepsy, mental illness, sensory impairment or increased likelihood of choking – all of which are more common amongst people with learning disabilities'.

Mencap (2007, p. 19) highlighted that 'the Disability Rights Commission (DRC) identified "diagnostic overshadowing" as a key barrier to people with a learning disability getting equal treatment'. Diagnostic overshadowing occurs when health care professionals 'wrongly believe that a presenting problem is a feature of someone's disability and that not much can be done about it. This can often lead to a wrong or no diagnosis of a medical condition that needs treatment'.

When you add to this the fact that many health care professionals often have limited experience of working with people with a learning disability, a lack of training in learning disability practice, and a lack of knowledge of their specific health care needs, it is no surprise that a hospital admission creates anxiety for the person, their family/carers and the health care professionals involved. A number of research projects and reports over the past 15 years have identified and highlighted these issues (*see 'Summary of current evidence base in Chapter 1'*).

Two of the key points to come from this evidence base are:

1. In comparison with the general population, people with learning disabilities have higher health needs with greater admissions to hospital but are known to have shorter episodes of care (Morgan 2000) cited in Brown (2005).

General Hospital Care for People with Learning Disabilities, First Edition by Lynn Hannon and Julie Clift
© 2011 Blackwell Publishing Ltd

2. Twenty-six per cent of people with learning disabilities are admitted to general hospitals each year in comparison to 14% of the general population, with families often feeling a need to 'take responsibility' for their dependants' care (Mencap 1998).

It is clear then that people with a learning disability are more likely to be admitted to hospital than the general population, and that general hospital services need to make 'reasonable adjustments' to ensure equal access to the health care they require to meet their needs.

It is also important to point out that whilst family/carers should not be expected to 'take responsibility', they should be actively involved at every stage of the patient journey. The 10-year Carers' Strategy, *Carers at the Heart of 21st Century Families and Communities* (2008) clearly sets out that carers are expected to be seen as full partners in the health care process, and should be involved in the diagnosis, provision of health care and discharge planning, working alongside the health care professionals.

HFT (2009, P. 4) highlight three key points which are central to many of the recommendations made in recent reports:

1. Like everyone else, people with learning disabilities should get the help they need from health services, though this may mean that reasonable adjustments need to be made.
2. health care professionals should listen more to the families and support staff of people with learning disabilities because they usually know most about them and the support they need.
3. Health staff should not rely on relatives or paid carers of people with learning disabilities to provide care whilst they are in hospital without considering their needs and supporting them appropriately.

The following diagram illustrates a typical patient journey through general hospital care and highlights the key health care professionals involved at each stage (Fig. 2.1).

- The learning disability (LD) nurse is a member of the Primary Health Care Team and often the health care professional who can coordinate initial access to health services for people with a learning disability. They could also offer support to the individual and their family/carers throughout the patient journey.
- The acute liaison nurse is usually an LD nurse with a specific remit to liaise and work with general hospital services to support and coordinate the process of health care for people with a learning disability admitted to hospital. They offer specific support to everyone involved in the patient journey and in particular provide advice and guidance to health care professionals working in the general hospital.

(See Chapter 6 for further detail of these roles.)

THE PATIENT JOURNEY

There are numerous models that health care professionals may use to approach the process of health care. For the purpose of illustration we will describe a model used for nursing intervention, though this could be adapted for any group of health care professionals.

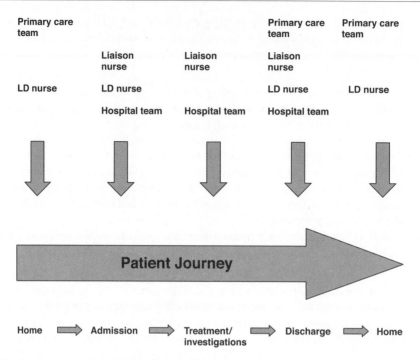

Fig. 2.1   Health care professional coordination of the patient's journey.

The 'nursing process' still provides the essential model for nursing intervention throughout the patient journey:

Assess, plan, implement, and evaluate

The assessment and planning typically take place prior to admission, and again at the point of admission. The implementation of health care takes place during admission, and the evaluation at the point of discharge, and in the time following a return to home. In practice, these steps are also ongoing and interchangeable throughout the process.

The Royal College of Nursing (RCN 2002) gives the core definition of nursing as 'The use of clinical judgement and the provision of care to enable people to promote, improve, maintain or recover health or, when death is inevitable, to die peacefully'. They describe the purpose of nursing as 'to promote health, healing, and normal growth and development; to prevent illness; and, when people become ill, to minimise distress and suffering, and to enable them to understand and cope with their disease, its treatment and its consequences'. This definition, describing the process of health care, could also be considered applicable to other groups of health professionals.

In order to explore the patient journey in more detail, we will consider the process of health care in general hospital services through the following points of access:

1. Accident and emergency department
2. Outpatients departments

3. Elective admission – medical
4. Elective admission – surgical

Accident and emergency department

The accident and emergency department is very likely to be the first point of access for many people to the hospital service. Cooper et al. (2004), therefore, suggest that it is imperative that the health care workers in this environment are able to 'identify patients that have learning disabilities and, in order to respond to the health needs of the patient, are able to appreciate the differing pattern of health disease experienced by this group'. Brown (2005) suggested that partnership working with specialists in learning disabilities health and emergency care can help to improve care.

During an emergency admission, it may be suspected that the patient has learning disabilities due to their presentation or communication abilities. Establishing that a person has a learning disability is not always an easy process, but speaking to the person or their carer (if present), to identify if they have any specific needs that should be taken into account, will ease the process of assessment, treatment, and if required, admission to hospital. (*See guidance in Chapter 1 on how to establish if your patient has a learning disability.*)

Initial assessment in the accident and emergency department usually takes place through the 'Triage' process and involves obtaining information from the individual in order to make an initial diagnosis. Triage is the allocation of clinical priority. The Manchester Triage Group (1997) suggests that clinical priority requires that enough information is gathered to enable the patient to be placed into one of the five categories defined in the National Triage Scale:

1. Identify the problem
2. Gather and analyse the information related to the solution
3. Evaluate all the alternatives and select one for implementation
4. Implement the selected alternative
5. Monitor the implementation and evaluate outcomes

Reflective Learning Point:

What would your priorities be if you were asked to triage a person with a learning disability admitted to your area of work and what factors could influence this process?

Determining the presenting condition and formulating a diagnosis is the primary function of triage, and this relies heavily on the reporting of the history of the condition and symptoms. It also relies on an ability to describe the nature and intensity of pain.

Process of Health Care Case Study 1 – Accident and Emergency

Jack is 48 years old. He has severe learning disabilities and autism. Jack fell up the stair when coming into the house. His care staff looked him over and noticed that he had cut his head, so took him to the emergency department at the local hospital. At the emergency department, he was assessed and received treatment for the laceration on his head.

Before leaving the emergency department, his care staff raised concerns that Jack was not his usual self. Jack had some obsessional behaviours that staff had noticed he was not doing. Jack always touches the top of the doorframe with his right hand when he walks through. Jack was looking at the frame but not raising his hand. Jack, who is usually very quiet, was vocalising a very low humming noise.

The care staff informed the doctor of this change in behaviour and he was examined further. Jack was found to have a fracture to his right clavicle. Jack was given pain relief and his arm was put into a support.

This case study illustrates the importance of health care professionals observing the non-verbal indicators (*see also Chapter 3*), discussing these with the individual and his family/carer, and the importance of taking into account of advice from someone who knows the person best.

When assessing patients with a learning disability pain cannot always be determined by self-reporting measures, such as analogue pain scales – which is the usual method and considered the most accurate guide on the patient's pain experience. There is evidence as described by Davis and Evans (2001) that some people with a learning disability do not present in the expected manner to pain, even though the pain may be acute. Therefore, pain assessment of the client group requires a skilled approach. (*For further information and guidance on pain assessment, see Chapter 4.*)

Admission to a receiving ward

When a patient with a learning disability has been admitted via the accident and emergency department, the nurse should attempt to identify a main carer and make contact with them as soon as possible in the patient's admission process to the acute hospital if this has not already been done. A full assessment of the patient's nursing needs should be undertaken. This will assist to identify the specific nursing resource required and should be done, if possible, in conjunction with the main carer.

Although some people with a learning disability may have paid or unpaid carers who will be able to give support at key times during the admission, it is rare that this support will be available 24 hours per day. In some circumstances, the commissioned carer may not be able to be in attendance at all. It is important that an agreement is negotiated early in the admission between the ward and the carer regarding the level of support need to be required. This can be tricky, especially when carers want to be in attendance at times that may not be convenient. By clearly identifying what support is needed at key points in the day a plan for support times can be made.

Often carers are concerned for the safety of the patient who may be distressed by the carer leaving and may try to wander from the ward. Equally, the ward staff may be anxious that they will be unable to identify the needs of a patient whose carers normally interpret the person's needs. Although these concerns are often valid, they are also often exaggerated by the anxiety of the unfamiliar environment. Continuous assessment of the patient need with consultation with the carer can usually help to minimise these anxieties and often no additional support is required. Any resource requirements that are identified should be communicated to the appropriate person as soon as possible and the necessary support instituted without delay.

By the very nature of an accident or emergency, the visit to hospital is not planned and this places a particular emphasis on health care professionals working in this area to have a working knowledge of the health needs of people with a learning disability with particular consideration of:

- Communication
- Behaviour
- Consent

(*See detailed guidance in relevant chapters for each of these areas.*)

The prior development of links with other professionals (such as LD nurses) who can help and are available to contact at the time of admission will greatly assist this process.

The following flowchart provides a template for the process of health care for a person with a learning disability during an emergency admission (Fig. 2.2).

Outpatient departments

Where a person is to attend for their first outpatient appointment they should, along with their carer/health facilitator, be invited to make advance contact with the clinic staff to discuss details of the nature of the appointment and to identify any special needs, for example access requirements, support needed for communication etc. This may also include a pre-appointment visit just to look around and become familiar with the clinic environment, and perhaps to meet staff who will be present on the day. Consideration should also be given to the carer and any support they may need, for example help with transport, help needed to explain any procedures, language difficulties etc.

One of the key factors that can help in outpatient departments is flexibility with clinic appointment times. Consideration should be given to the person's normal daily routine and if possible arrange appointments that may cause minimal disruption to this routine. If the person is likely to find waiting difficult, for example, due to behavioural needs, it will help greatly to offer them the first appointment on the day. This will also help to reduce any anxiety that may be created just from being in the hospital environment, and avoid any further distress for the individual or other patients. It may also be useful to consider using single rooms for the appointment and access to the clinic through quiet areas rather than passing through busy waiting areas. Where a person is a regular attendee at the clinic, it is beneficial if the same staff can be involved in the health care process as this helps them to develop a good understanding of the individual and their needs, and increases staff confidence in supporting the individual in the clinic.

Following the outpatient appointment a health care professional should check with the individual and their carer/health facilitator that they have understood everything that was discussed, what it meant, and what (if anything) is going to happen next. This should also include information about any further health care interventions that may be needed.

Any specific factors that help with the appointment should be recorded on the patient record for future reference, and the more of the health care process that can be planned in advance the more likely it is to be successful on the day.

Case study 2 outlines the simple adjustments that can be made to improve the experience for the patient in the outpatient department.

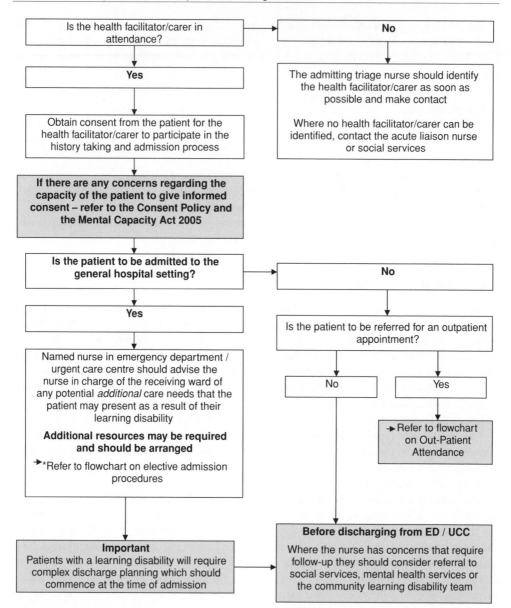

Fig. 2.2   Emergency admission. Reproduced with permission from Staffordshire and Shropshire PCT/A2A Network.

Process of Health Care Case Study 2 – Outpatients Department

Sheila is a regular patient at the rheumatology clinic. She likes her own company and tends to sit in her own area at home away from other family members. She does not like attending because she finds it difficult sitting in the waiting area with the other patients. She will scream loudly and try to run from the waiting area.

The nurse leading the clinic arranges for Sheila to be able to sit in a side room where she is able to sit at a desk and enjoy a jigsaw while she waits for her turn. Her parents bring her a selection of activities in case there is a delay. Sheila usually attends for the first appointment of the day to minimise the length of time she has to wait.

The doctor comes to the room where Sheila is waiting because she finds this less stressful. Sometimes she needs to have a blood test so these are taken by the clinic nurse while she is waiting so that she does not have to go to another area to have this procedure.

By minimising the movement of Sheila around the outpatients, department allows her to remain in a calm and receptive mood which allows her to access the health care assessment she requires.

The following flowchart provides a template for the process of health care for a person with a learning disability during an outpatient attendance (Fig. 2.3).

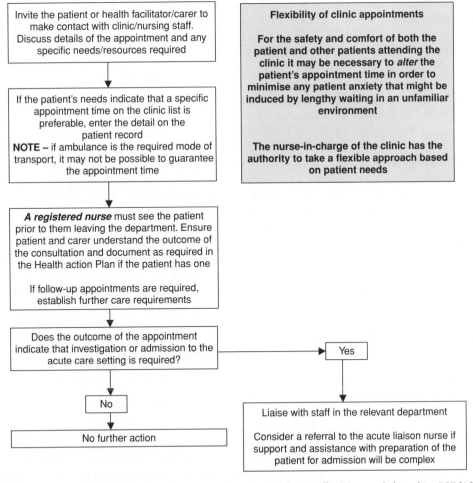

Fig. 2.3 Outpatient attendance. Reproduced with permission from staffordshire and shropshire PCT/A2A Network.

Elective admission – medical

When a person with a learning disability is to have a planned admission to hospital, this provides the opportunity to undertake an in-depth assessment of the individual needs in advance of the admission, and develop a person-centred plan for the health care process required. It is important that this happens as soon as a planned admission is agreed and, where the person's needs may be complex, the LD nurse or acute liaison nurse will be able to offer specific advice and support throughout the process.

Where information is available in advance the health care professional who will be responsible for the department should be informed that a person with a learning disability is to be admitted and should be provided with contact details of the carer/health facilitator. A named person should be identified who will be on duty and take responsibility for the individual on the day of admission, and the LD nurse or acute liaison nurse should be contacted for information on whether the person is known to health or social services.

The key to a successful planned admission is the pre-admission part of the health care process. (The pre-admission process is explored in much more detail later in this chapter.) Where possible, a pre-admission visit to the ward/department can be really valuable. It provides the ideal opportunity for hospital staff to meet the individual and for the individual to become familiar with the hospital environment. It allows time to explore individual needs and consider/identify any additional resources that may be needed to support the admission.

It is important to highlight that any care needs that the individual has are the responsibility of hospital staff during the admission.

Carers/families should not be expected to provide care for the individual though they will provide valuable support and advice for the hospital staff. They should be invited to accompany the person on the day of admission and take part in the admission process with them. They should also be actively involved in planning the care of the person. Some carers may wish to contribute to the care of the person and, even though this is a voluntary action, they should be supported to do this where appropriate.

On the day of admission a full nursing assessment should be carried out using the ward's usual nursing model/standard assessment tool. This should be combined with any additional assessments undertaken as part of the pre-admission assessment process. The expertise of the LD nurse and/or acute liaison nurse can be particularly useful in undertaking a thorough and detailed assessment. They will also have access to specific assessment tools, for example around communication or behavioural needs, which would not be generally available.

The following case study illustrates a simple planned admission process:

Process of Health Care Case Study 3 – Elective Admission (Medical)

Andrew is due to be admitted to hospital for chemotherapy as part of his ongoing treatment for non-Hodgkin lymphoma. Andrew has a current 'Prior to Hospital Admission Assessment' that informs the heath care staff of Andrew's needs. Prior to coming into hospital Andrew visits the ward with his carer and the LD liaison nurse to introduce himself to the ward team and to discuss the admission. Together they identify key times in the day when Andrew will need support from his carer so that he can be there to support him. Andrew uses Makaton to communicate his needs so they bring a communication book for the ward staff with some of his signs.

On the day of the admission the nurse Andrew met on his visit is able to complete his admission assessment which includes the information from Andrew's prior to admission assessment.

(Makaton is a form of sign language especially devised for people with learning disabilities. For more information, see Chapter 3 or visit: www.makaton.org.uk.)

Health care professionals working in partnership with people who know Andrew well ensured his specific needs were identified and met, and contributed to a successful admission to hospital.

The following flowchart provides a template for the process of health care for a person with a learning disability during an elective admission (Fig. 2.4).

Elective admission – surgical

The advice for elective admission (medical) as outlined in the previous section should be followed for a surgical admission, and further consideration should be given to the additional factors of pre-operative preparation (including pain assessment and management), anaesthesia and recovery. Carer support is also important to facilitate a successful admission.

Health care staff from the person's ward should contact the theatre staff at least 24 hours in advance to ensure they are aware that they will be receiving someone with a learning disability and to discuss any specific health needs this may present. This information should also be passed on to the recovery team. A pre-operative visit should have been planned in advance (during pre-admission stage) in order to identify any special needs, for example access requirements, support needed for communication etc. The carer/health facilitator may be invited to accompany the person to the theatre suite with the ward nurse.

The following pre-operative preparation issues should be discussed with the individual and their carer/health facilitator:

- The person's previous experience of anaesthesia and surgery
- Any known behavioural patterns which may become evident when the person recovers from the anaesthetic state
- The person's communication needs
- Whether the carer/health facilitator wishes to accompany the person to the anaesthetic room and/or be present in the recovery room
- Whether a ward nurse needs to stay with the person in the anaesthetic room until they are asleep to provide continuity of care and support

Particular consideration must be given to pain assessment and management with a pre-operative visit by the pain team to discuss this issue with the individual, their carer/health facilitator and ward staff. People with a learning disability may communicate pain differently and individual pain assessment techniques should be implemented to ensure adequate pain management. The theatre care plan should be used to document the person's needs in both the anaesthetic and recovery rooms.

Sister/Charge nurse to be informed **in advance** by nursing, medical and/or secretarial staff of the patient's:
1. Clinical needs
2. Admission date
3. Health facilitator/carer

Instructions
Consider how the patient needs to be informed of the treatment.
The information must be in an accessible format suitable for the individual
For example, on audio tape, in pictures or photographs
The acute liaison nurse can help with this

↓

Sister/Charge nurse to identify a **named nurse** and ensure that they are on duty on the day of the patient's admission

↓

Named nurse to **make contact with patient and health facilitator/carer** prior to admission to:
- Invite them to attend the ward prior to admission for familiarisation
- Discuss admission arrangements
- Discuss current care needs and specific equipment
- Seek consent for carer involvement during admission
- Negotiate carer and ward staff roles
- To identify any additional nursing resources required
- Suggest referral to acute liaison nurse

Medications
Specific attention should be given to the patient's medication regime including preparation, times and method of administration; these will have been tailored to the individual patient's needs and should continue while in hospital

↓

If the patient assessment identifies that the patient requires additional nursing support discuss with the Matron and arrange additional resources?

↓

Day of admission
- A full nursing and medical assessment is undertaken
- If the health facilitator/carer is unable to be involved in the admission process then ascertain contact and document
- Where the patient attends without a health facilitator/carer, with the patient's consent the nurse should make a carer relative or social services aware of the patient's admission

→

Discharge planning
Patients with a learning disability have **complex discharge planning needs**

Discharge planning should be discussed at the time of admission. The discharge co-ordinator and acute liaison nurse can arrange appropriate referrals e.g., assistance with independent living, district nurse, GP.

Fig. 2.4   Elective admission. Reproduced with permission from staffordshire and shropshire PCT/A2A Network.

(For further information and guidance on communication, see Chapter 3 and on pain assessment, see Chapter 4.)

The use of anaesthesia and the effect of this should be clearly explained to the individual in a way that they can understand wherever possible. Their level of understanding should be clarified with their carer/health facilitator and any issues relating to compliance with the procedure should be discussed. Where a procedure is to take place under a local anaesthetic it may be appropriate for the carer/health facilitator to remain with the person throughout the procedure.

It may sometimes be appropriate to use a general anaesthetic where a person's ability to tolerate or cooperate with a procedure is unclear. For example, to undertake an MRI scan, though the use of desensitisation processes (*see later section in this chapter on intervention and treatment*) should be considered first.

If the carer/health facilitator is to be present in the recovery room, arrangements should be made for how they are to be contacted, and wherever possible, the recovery nurse/ward nurse known to the person should transfer them back to the ward.

Process of Health Care Case Study 4 – Elective Admission (Surgical)

Charles is 60 and has Down's syndrome. His care staff had noticed a lump in his groin that they reported to his general practitioner (GP). Charles has refused to have any physical examinations in the past so his GP referred on to a surgeon at the hospital for advice.

The surgeon came to see Charles at home and took the opportunity of observing the lump while he was dressing. The surgeon agreed that this was a hernia and that it would be in Charles's best interest to remove it.

The care staff were concerned that they would not be able to get Charles to the hospital for surgery as they had not been able to get Charles to attend the GP surgery. The acute liaison nurse visited Charles at home to establish how he could be prepared to go into hospital for the surgery.

The nurse assessed that Charles had very little comprehension and was unable to understand why he needed to go into hospital. Neither could he inform the nurse of why he did not like to go to the doctor's surgery.

The nurse talked with the care staff about Charles's interests and likes and dislikes. They established that Charles likes to spend his time looking through magazines, drinking tea, going to cafes and listening to Tom Jones. He did not like unfamiliar people, being undressed – except when it is bedtime, and not having buttons on his cardigan.

A plan was devised to help build Charles's confidence entering the hospital so they could arrange for him to come to day surgery to have his hernia repair.

The care staff brought Charles up to the hospital canteen for his lunch as an introduction to the hospital environment. They then started visiting the day surgery reception where he had a cup of tea and the opportunity to look through the magazines. During this time he met with the nursing team and the anaesthetist was able to see him. Charles made several visits to the day surgery department. He was gradually introduced to the ward area and had the opportunity to sit on the bed.

The care staff helped the nursing staff to pick up on the clues that Charles was unhappy. If feeling unsure Charles would pick at the buttons on his cardigan and he would move as to go to the car if he was feeling threatened.

As Charles's confidence grew the nursing staff were able to introduce him to equipment until he was happy to let the nurse take his blood pressure.

Prior to the date for admission the care staff and the pre-operative nurse made a plan for the day. Charles would be first on the theatre list. He would attend with two staff who knew him well, and the nurses on duty on the day surgery department had also spent some time getting to know him, and how to help manage Charles's anxiety. They would have a Tom Jones CD to distract him and a selection of new magazines.

This example highlights the importance of partnership working; with each person involved having a vital part to play in what was a successful admission. It also demonstrates how person-centred assessment and care planning form the basis for the process of health care to take place, with reasonable adjustments being made to enable the individual to access the health care he needed.

The following flowchart provides a template for the process of health care for a person with a learning disability attending theatre and recovery (Fig. 2.5).

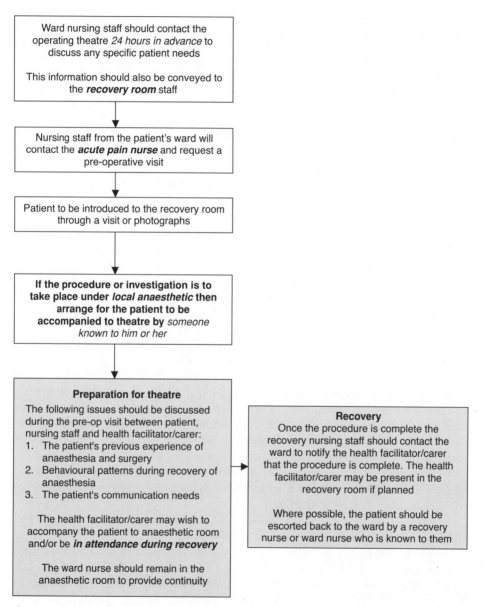

Fig. 2.5 Patients attending theatre and recovery. Reproduced with permission from staffordshire and shropshire PCT/A2A Network.

PRE-ADMISSION

People with a learning disability are often vulnerable and frightened when admitted to hospital. Health care professionals who are aware of and sensitive to their individual needs can contribute greatly to making the admission a positive experience. It is also important to fully involve families/carers, and other people who know that person, and consider how they can pass on their knowledge to hospital staff to support them to care for that person whilst in hospital, and reduce pressure on the carer. The pre-admission process provides the ideal opportunity for this to take place.

The main organisational advantages of pre-admission assessment include:

- Time to undertake comprehensive assessments prior to admission
- Opportunity to pre-plan care and discharge to ensure efficient use of resources and the potential for reducing numbers of cancelled operations or blocked beds
- Can contribute to shorter length of stay in hospital
- Health promotion can begin at the pre-admission stage
- Quality of overall health care process is improved

It is important at pre-admission to establish the diagnosis of the learning disability which may sometimes highlight complications related to a particular condition. (*See Chapter 1 for further information about causes of learning disability.*) It is also important that health care professionals do not stereotype people just because of their condition, for example people with Down's syndrome may sometimes be easy to recognise but can greatly differ in terms of their individual ability levels and needs.

The pre-admission assessment and care planning process should begin as soon as it is known that a person with a learning disability requires a hospital admission. The in-depth assessment should establish the person's individual needs in advance of the admission. The process should involve the individual, their carer/health facilitator, hospital staff and, where appropriate, an LD nurse or acute liaison nurse. Other health care professionals involved with the person, for example the speech and language therapists are also able to provide a valuable contribution.

The pre-admission assessment should take into account of the individual's physical, psychological, social and cultural needs and how these can be met during the hospital admission. This may well be different from how these needs are usually met in their home environment. For a person with a learning disability the assessment of the additional areas of consent, behaviour and communication needs should also form a part of this process.

HFT (2009, p. 20) highlights the importance of the need to share information and discuss the following:

- The presenting medical need, including treatment required and how this will be carried out
- Expected outcome and possible areas of risk
- Communication aids or communication patterns to be explained to hospital staff so that they are aware of the ways the person expresses themselves
- The person's likely reactions to the hospital environment and procedures – will restraint be necessary? And how is this best delivered?
- Whether or not the person should be resuscitated if a cardiac arrest occurs

Particular note should be made of the person's medication regime, including the form of the preparation, times and methods of administration, which could be very specific to each individual.

Your local LD nurse or acute liaison nurse will probably have examples of a standard pre-admission assessment tool that they can use. The following is an example template of a pre-admission assessment tool which you may wish to consider:

NHS

East Lancashire Community Services

COMMUNITY-BASED ASSESSMENT FOR PEOPLE WITH LEARNING DISABILITIES – PRIOR TO HOSPITAL ADMISSION

Name:

DoB:

Important things you need to know about me:

People involved in assessment

NAME	ROLE

Date completed:

Date of admission:

Hospital Ward/Department:

Acknowledgements: Lothian University Hospital NHS Trust
Lothian Primary Care NHS Trust
West Hampshire NHS Trust

Assessment Rating Scale: (Level of support required)
(*areas scoring 2–4 must have Health Action Plan completed)

Score:	0	No support required, capable of safe, independent care
	1	Appropriate support can be provided by ward
	2	Appropriate additional support can be provided by family or existing paid carers
	3	Additional ward support will be required
	4	Additional support from specialist paid support staff is required

Risk Assessment Rating:

Low	No or low risk of impact on admission
Medium	Likely risk of impact on admission
High	Very likely that there will be impact on admission

COMMUNICATION *(What is the best way to communicate with the person, verbal, non-verbal, signs, gestures, noises, words commonly used and meanings, what is the person most likely to communicate about, how would they indicate pain?)*

Score:

Risk:
Low
Medium
High

SKILLS *(What is the person able to do relating to personal care, what help is needed?)*

Score:

Risk:
Low
Medium
High

EATING AND DRINKING *(What does the person use for eating/drinking, any aids, special diets, likes and dislikes, swallowing difficulties etc?)*

Score:

Risk:
Low
Medium
High

CONTINENCE *(Does the person use continence aids, any help needed?)*

Score:

Risk:
Low
Medium
High

MOBILITY *(Does the person use aids, support needed with certain tasks etc.?)*	**Score:**
	Risk: **Low** **Medium** **High**

MEDICATION *(How does the person take medication e.g. spoon, syringe, with food etc.?)*	**Score:**
	Risk: **Low** **Medium** **High**

SLEEP PATTERN *(Usual bedtimes, how long does the person usually sleep, any routines, any problems or sleep disturbances?)*	**Score:**
	Risk: **Low** **Medium** **High**

BEHAVIOUR *(Does the person display any unusual behaviours, are there any triggers, how do carers deal with these behaviours?)*	**Score:**
	Risk: **Low** **Medium** **High**

ASSOCIATED CONDITIONS *(Any conditions staff should be aware of e.g. epilepsy, specific syndromes, how is this condition managed, any specific guidelines for practice?)*	**Score:**
	Risk: **Low** **Medium** **High**

LIKES AND DISLIKES *(For all aspects of the person's life e.g. food, drink, occupation/activities, people, environment?)*	<u>Score:</u>
	<u>Risk</u>: Low Medium High

MENTAL HEALTH NEEDS *(Any specific diagnosis, approaches/additional support needed, interventions?)*	<u>Score:</u>
	<u>Risk</u>: Low Medium High

SAFETY/RISK ISSUES *(Level of awareness of environment, safety of self and others)*	<u>Score:</u>
	<u>Risk</u>: Low Medium High

USUAL DAILY ROUTINE *(What is usual routine, will being in hospital distress the person, will routine be affected after discharge, will lifestyle affect treatment given?)*	<u>Score:</u>
	<u>Risk</u>: Low Medium High

FAMILY/CARER NEEDS *(During hospital admission and following discharge)*	<u>Score:</u>
	<u>Risk</u>: Low Medium High

HEALTH CARE PROCEDURES *(Specific procedures during this admission, help needed for explanation, preparation, planning, co-operation)*	**Score:**
	Risk: Low Medium High

CONSENT ISSUES *(How is consent given e.g. written, verbal, implied, best interests, any areas of concern?)*	**Score:**
	Risk: Low Medium High

ANY OTHER ISSUES	**Score:**
	Risk: Low Medium High

COMMENTS

HEALTH ACTION PLAN
(Based on pre-admission assessment of needs)

NAME:				

Areas of Need Identified	Action Needed	Person(s) Responsible	Needs Met	Needs Unmet

Comments:	
Health Action Plan completed by:	
Date:	

HFT guidance (2009) includes a template for two other types of assessment: the Traffic Light Hospital Assessment and the Risk, Dependency and Support Assessment for patients with a learning disability. Whatever tool is used should provide the hospital staff with useful information about the individual to assist with the planning and provision of health care.

A copy of the HFT (2009) report 'Working Together: Easy Steps to Improving How People with a Learning Disability Are Supported When in Hospital' can be downloaded from: http://www.hft.org.uk/p/4/121/Working_Together.html *or* http://valuingpeople.gov.uk/dynamic/valuingpeople118.jsp.

A named health care professional should be identified who will take lead responsibility for the individual on the day of admission. Ideally the lead health care professional should meet the person before admission, perhaps arranging a visit to the ward/department in order to carry out the detailed assessment. This provides a good opportunity to meet the health professionals involved, find out about car parking, bathrooms, ward areas, dining arrangements and other services that may be available. It is also important at this point to identify any additional resources that may be required during the admission.

The person and their carer will need to be supported to understand why they are going into hospital and what is going to happen to them. This may involve the use of communication aids, for example pictures or photographs to illustrate procedures or equipment. (*See further information in Chapter 3.*)

The evidence base (see Chapter 1) highlights a range of problems associated with hospital admissions for people with a learning disability. A project team in Edinburgh was among the first group of professionals to introduce initiatives designed to address the problems reported. Brown and MacArthur (1999) were part of a team of acute and community learning disability nursing services who worked together to develop a framework for assessing and supporting people with learning disabilities in the acute setting.

They designed the original Dependency Assessment Scale, which was a pre-admission assessment tool designed to identify the level of support a person with a learning disability needed during their hospital admission. They also introduced a hospital liaison nurse role within the learning disability team. These interventions were designed to facilitate a person-centred approach, including individual assessment of needs and care planning, which took into account any adjustments needed to the process of health care. Both interventions showed positive benefits when reviewed after 3 years.

Looking at wider research conducted with comparable groups, Davis and Marsden (2001) evaluated a newly established post of clinical nurse specialist (CNS) for disabled people in a large general hospital. The study mainly involved people with physical disabilities, but also included a number of people with learning disabilities.

The key elements of the role involved pre-admission assessment of needs relating to the disability, preparation of personal plans, liaison with relevant wards, organisation of equipment etc. prior to admission, and working with staff in the acute area to give them support and confidence in dealing with the individual. A programme of disability awareness raising seminars, attitude assessment and team meetings were also carried out.

The study concluded that some disabled people were not having their needs met in hospital, and the main reason for this was a lack of awareness among staff about disability issues. Nurses focused on the disability rather than the individual. The CNS role was seen as valuable and had positive benefits for both people with disabilities and hospital staff, and interventions were seen as very effective.

Factors to consider in the pre-admission process

The purpose of the pre-admission assessment meeting is to clarify the health care process, identify the individual's needs and agree all of the arrangements for the actual admission.

The key factors to consider in the pre-admission meeting are:

- The individual and their specific care needs, as identified from any assessment tool used or information shared
- What the person can do for themselves
- What they will need help with and any additional resources that may be required
- The environment they will be in and any adjustments that may be needed to accommodate their needs
- The intervention they are being admitted for and what procedures need to be carried out
- Carers' needs, including active involvement and support of carers in the health care process
- Any risk issues (e.g. behaviour, vulnerability, safeguarding issues)
- Consent, the individual's capacity to consent, and how consent is to be obtained
- How the person communicates and any aids to communication that may be needed, including how to enable the person to understand what is going to happen to them
- Identify the lead health care professional with responsibility for the person during their hospital admission, and contact details for other key people involved
- Clarify roles and 'who will do what'
- Discharge planning should also be considered at this point in the health care process

To comply with equality and diversity legislation such as the Disability Discrimination Act (DDA; 1995), all hospitals should have a 'disability equality scheme', though in practice this is often incorporated into a 'single equality scheme'. HFT (2009) states that hospitals have a clear 'duty of equality'. This does not mean treating everybody the same but rather that hospitals must make 'reasonable adjustments' to meet the needs of disabled people, because they are entitled to expect equality in the outcome of their hospital stay.

HFT (2009) suggests a number of steps that families/carers can undertake to prepare for hospital admissions (planned or unplanned) such as:

- Collecting together information about the person and their specific needs. This may be in the form of an assessment, person-centred care plan or health action plan (HAP) (*see later section on Care Planning for further information about HAP*)
- Consider any advance decisions (e.g. about resuscitation)
- Collect together information about people who may be able to help with a hospital admission (e.g. the acute liaison nurse, PALS)
- Identify any particular support that may be needed in hospital and who will provide this
- Identify any potential capacity or consent issues

They provide a useful list (p. 21) of possible questions for the pre-admission meeting that have been suggested by family members, such as:

- Are drinks offered to relatives when they are beside patients or should they take their own refreshments?
- Should you take special spoons/cups or does the ward have them?

- Does the hospital provide accommodation for carers providing additional support?
- Specialist equipment needs – does the hospital have things like hoists, accessible baths etc.?

They also suggest steps for hospitals to prepare for the admission of patients with a learning disability which are covered in the later section on Care Planning and developing Care Pathways.

A copy of the HFT (2009) report 'Working Together: Easy Steps to Improving How People with a Learning Disability Are Supported When in Hospital' can be downloaded from: http://www.hft.org.uk/p/4/121/Working_Together.html *or* http://valuingpeople.gov.uk/dynamic/valuingpeople118.jsp.

Benefits of pre-admission assessment

Hannon (2003) undertook a research project where she designed and introduced a standard pre-admission assessment tool to be used when people with a learning disability were being admitted to hospital.

The primary aim for the study was to:

- Explore the experience of the health care process from the perspective of four different stakeholders; the person with a learning disability, their family/carers, hospital staff and community learning disability nurses.

The specific objectives were to:

- Identify key factors that influence the process of health care
- Evaluate the impact of the pre-admission assessment tool
- Compare results of this study with the current evidence base

A qualitative research approach was taken as a way of developing knowledge of the health care process. Ploeg (1999) describes the purpose of qualitative research as 'to describe, explore, and explain phenomena being studied. Qualitative research questions often take the form of what is this, or what is happening here, and are more concerned with the process than the outcome'.

A qualitative approach was taken for a number of reasons including:

- Limited knowledge available about the topic area
- The study explores the personal experience of the stakeholders
- Study is concerned with the process of health care
- The exploratory and diagnostic nature of study
- A qualitative approach is more suited to facilitate participation of service users
- Research is conducted with rather than on people

The study involved a process evaluation with multiple stakeholder analysis. Methods chosen for data collection were a focus group and semi-structured interviews. Standard questions were prepared in advance and used for all participants. Øvretveit (1998, p. 43) outlines the aim of process evaluations as, 'to give people an understanding of how a service operates and of how the service produces what it does'. This is useful where you want to know why something is effective.

Box 2.1 Key Features of Framework Analysis

Grounded or generative: it is heavily based in, and driven by, the original accounts and observations of the people it is about.

Dynamic: it is open to change, addition and amendment throughout the analytic process.

Systematic: it allows methodical treatment of all similar units of analysis.

Comprehensive: it allows a full, and not partial or selective, review of the material collected.

Enables easy retrieval: it allows access to, and retrieval of, the original textual material.

Allows between-case and within-case analysis: it enables comparisons between, and associations within, cases to be made.

Accessible to others: the analytic process, and the interpretations derived from it, can be viewed and judged by people other than the primary analyst.

A multiple, typical case, convenience sample was identified. The population targeted and the inclusion criteria were people with a learning disability, within community nurse caseload, with a planned hospital admission. Service user participants represented a range of ability levels, from mild to severe learning disability and included communication and behaviour problems, as these are both highlighted in the evidence base. The researcher remained independent of the health care process.

Data analysis in qualitative research is essentially inductive; that is, the findings emerge from the data collected and are not pre-determined. A 'framework' approach was used by Ritchie and Spencer (1993) for analysis within the study.

Framework enables analysis in four categories:

- *Contextual:* identifying the form and nature of what exists.
- *Diagnostic:* examining the reasons for, or causes of, what exists.
- *Evaluative:* appraising the effectiveness of what exists.
- *Strategic:* identifying new theories, policies, plans or actions.

The key features of this method are summarised in Box 2.1.

Evaluation of the impact of pre-admission assessment

The hypothesis of the study was that there is a positive causal relationship between the use of a standard pre-admission assessment and improved outcomes for people with a learning disability admitted for general hospital care. Analysis is in the format of responses received from each stakeholder group to the assessment. This is intended to enable clearer triangulation of the data.

Note that the reference numbers in [ ] brackets refer to the data reference from the interview transcript. All names are fictitious to maintain confidentiality.

Service user responses

When a carer explained purpose of the assessment to Alan, despite his limited verbal skills, he said [2.374] 'That's a good idea' very loud and clear.

Lucy was pleased that staff knew what she needed [11.76] 'Because (community nurse) told them'.

Steven felt [20.438] 'It helped, by she described me what it was going to be like in there, so it made me at ease, so I would know what I was putting myself into'.

Family/carer's responses

Carers felt the pre-admission assessment gave them confidence in the hospital staff and reduced their anxiety. They valued being actively involved in the process and felt that it was important to highlight what the person could do and what they needed support with. The assessment identified the person's specific needs and enabled person-centred care planning to take place.

All carers felt it was important to help hospital staff understand how much the person could do for themselves, and what they needed support with.

Alan's carer commented [3.241] 'If they'd only take a few minutes just to read it they'd find looking after Alan much easier'. Mary's carer said [7.151] 'I think it was brilliant, brilliant yes'. [7.156] 'They knew what she was about; there weren't sort of any surprises round the corner'. Lucy's carer thought it was [14.59] 'Helpful for the person being admitted and for the staff'.

David's mum said [16.27] 'I think it just covered everything and it was in a format that you could read very easily'. [16.186] 'I just felt relaxed to go in without the added stress of explaining things to people when I am looking after a child at the same time'.

Hospital staff responses

Hospital staff felt better informed and prepared. They were able to cope with communication difficulties and complex behavioural problems because they knew what to expect and had received support prior to the admission.

Although Alan was well known to hospital staff, they found out things that they had not previously known, and thought the assessment was particularly useful for new staff to the ward.

For Mary, [8.109–113] 'With the pre-op assessment it gave us information about her set regime. We know that she needs less interrupting and that she likes tea'. [8.133] 'It's an excellent idea. Very, very good, because a lot of nurses like in a general hospital don't have experience in dealing with patients with learning disabilities, you know'.

Lucy's staff felt [10.100] 'It was very helpful, there's all this information I thought that's marvellous, at least we know that she wants these things and we were able to read about how she liked to do things and what she liked to do. It was very involved, very in-depth and thorough'. [10.205] 'If people are coming again and they have got this sort of care package set out it will be wonderful'.

David's staff noted that [15.19] 'With the children with special needs you tend to find that their notes are very, very thick and it can take a considerable amount of time to actually find out what they are capable or not capable of doing, and their normal responses. I found that all the information that I needed for looking after David was on that sheet'. [15.43–44] 'I could not believe the day went so well. It was so well organised, well planned and everybody knew what they were doing. It was all due to the information received beforehand. That we were ready, prepared'.

Hospital staff working with Steven said [18.123/129] 'I thought it was brilliant, and if everybody had information like that life would be a lot easier and quicker'.

Hospital staff found they were confident in caring for the person because they felt better informed, and prepared. They valued the support and input from the learning disability nurse.

Community LD nurse responses

The assessment took approximately 30–45 minutes to complete. All areas were relevant and nothing seemed to be missing. [17.122] 'The scoring made you focus on what were the important sections'.

The nurses highlighted that the way they wrote the assessment could help present a positive image of the person, even where there were problems identified. It helped focus the service user on what was going to happen and provided an opportunity to address any concerns.

Community nurses described the importance of preparing clients for admission, and of initial contact and preparation with hospital staff. They felt their presence reassured the other stakeholders, particularly one carer who also had a learning disability and felt nervous around professionals. The assessment included service users and carers in consultation, and was a valuable way of getting information across to the hospital staff. They felt hospital staff were able to prepare for areas of need identified, rather than finding out things just as a person was admitted.

Community nurses highlighted that some people with a learning disability appear more capable than they actually are, and that hospital staff have difficulty with making judgements about an individual's level of functioning.

Alan's community nurse said [1.82] 'I did wonder how I would sort of be able to just quickly get a Health Action Plan from it, then it just fell into place, really quickly' and [1.84] 'I think the main thing about it was just keeping it simple'.

They found hospital staff were pleased to accept the assessment and HAP from them. It was seen as straightforward and unambiguous, and enabled good liaison to take place.

Mary's community nurse said [5.270] 'I think that was the feeling I got that you know they (hospital staff) were happy to do it because they could see some benefits for themselves. They didn't see it as a paper exercise at all'. [5.163] 'If you're prepared you have a different mind set. You approach people in a different way'.

Lucy's community nurse said [9.171–175] 'I think it is an excellent thing to actually have available for myself as well as the client. I found it less stressful actually having this to work through. It can make their stay in hospital much better'. [9.136] 'The Health Action Plan at the end I thought was really good, because it was clear there as to what was pulled out of the assessment, and it's clear then as to what would make Lucy's stay in hospital better, and more comfortable for her'.

David's community nurse saw it as beneficial for his carer, [13.153–157] 'She was more secure because she knew the people knew about his needs. And it was all done for her, she didn't have to keep repeating, explaining or apologising for his behaviour because it had all been done'.

Steven's community nurse felt [17.128] 'They were reassured by that information because they had everything written down'. One community nurse commented [1.147] 'Yes, it formalises things perhaps we have tried to do in the past, but it makes it easier and it makes it one system'.

Key points from individual interview feedback

- People with a learning disability have a good understanding of their own health needs.
- LD nurses have a good understanding of the health needs of people with learning disabilities.
- Use of the pre-admission assessment had a positive effect on the health care process.
- There was good evidence of person-centred approaches to care planning, with care plans that were responsive to the needs of individuals.
- There was a high level of satisfaction with health care process across all stakeholder groups.
- People with learning disabilities felt they were treated the same as everyone else.

- Attitudes of hospital staff towards people with learning disabilities were more positive than expected.
- Hospital staff showed a positive attitude towards the role and input of LD nurses.
- Active liaison between services was welcomed, and very effective.
- Hospital staff identified that they need more training about learning disability issues.

Summary of impact of the pre-admission assessment

The nursing process – assess, plan, implement and evaluate – formed the basis of the health care process for all the individuals involved. Evaluation of admissions showed consistently high satisfaction rating scores, with good correlation across all stakeholder groups. A total of 100% of stakeholders rated health care as 'satisfactory' or above, with almost 70% rating it as 'excellent'.

For service users the assessment identified their individual and specific needs, and provided the basis for person-centred care planning to take place. Consultation and active involvement was a key element of the process. Service users said that the assessment is a good idea, it helps to explain things about them to hospital staff, helps with preparation for admission, identifies level of support needed, tells hospital staff what they like and puts people at ease. The assessment helped to focus care planning on the needs of the individual, and enabled valuable preparation to occur.

Carers felt hospital staff sometimes show a lack of understanding of the needs of people with learning disabilities, but within this study, they were happy with the support received, and health care provided. Carers felt that the assessment gave them confidence in the ability of hospital staff to care for the person because they were better informed as to what their needs were. It reduced their anxiety, and they valued being actively involved in the process. Carers felt more relaxed that it took some responsibility away from them for having to explain everything to hospital staff. They felt hospital staff had taken note of what the person needed, and were flexible in meeting the needs identified. Carers felt it important to highlight what the person could do for themselves and what they needed support with. This helps reduce potential for under/over-protection. They felt that the assessment is in an easy-to-read format, and includes everything that was needed.

Perhaps the most positive evaluations came from hospital staff. They felt they had particularly benefited by being better informed about the person and better prepared. Even communication and complex behaviour problems were coped with during the admission because they were supported, and knew what to expect.

Hospital staff thought the assessment had made all the difference. It is clear, and gave them easy access to everything they needed to know about that person. It saved them looking through reams of hospital notes, and addressed the issue of lack of understanding highlighted in the evidence base. It reduced their anxiety, and they were able to plan in advance, which increased their confidence in their ability to cope with the person. Initial fears were replaced by a much more positive attitude towards people with a learning disability. Hospital staff suggested there is potential for using a similar pre-admission assessment process for other groups of vulnerable people.

LD nurses thought the assessment worked well to identify service user needs, and help with their preparation for admission. The scoring system helped them to highlight the main areas of need. It is easy to read, included everything that was needed, was straightforward to use, not too time-consuming and enabled good liaison to take place. It provided a standard tool and a system to formalise things they have tried to do in the past. They found the assessment useful to prepare service user, carer and hospital staff. It helped them to focus on the admission and provided an opportunity to discuss any concerns. They thought it helped to make the stay in hospital better for the person, that carers felt more secure because everything was written down, and found it was a less stressful experience for them too.

Potentially the most problematic admission, of a person with autism, severe learning disability, no communication and very difficult behaviour, actually received the highest overall rating scores from stakeholders. The admission went like clockwork; hospital staff were prepared, flexible and responsive to his very complex needs. Active liaison and support was provided by the LD nurse, mum was relaxed, the service user was happy and his health needs were fully met. Everyone involved reported that this was due to the use of the assessment. A completely person-centred approach was taken to his care planning with excellent outcomes for everyone involved.

Process of Health Care Case Study 5 – Pre-Admission Assessment

Danny is an 8-year-old boy with autism, severe learning disability, limited communication and challenging behaviour. His mum stayed throughout the admission. She was anxious about this, as she had no previous experience of hospital admissions with him. His community nurse, who has 26 years of nursing experience, but has only known Danny for 4 months, visited them before the admission. The community nurse provided information for hospital staff about autism and behaviour management strategies.

The hospital staff caring for Danny had 22 years of experience as a children's nurse, and has cared for people with learning disabilities on a number of previous occasions.

A good deal of preparation had taken place by hospital staff in response to the information from the pre-admission assessment regarding Danny's specific needs. Mum noticed this and said [16.16] 'I felt that everything was prepared and ready for him'.

Whilst mum felt that people with a learning disability should be treated the same as everyone else she commented, [16.134–135] 'Sometimes they need to be treated differently because of their learning disability and I don't think that is always taken into account. I think sometimes they need that bit more care and attention'.

Mum thought it was the little things that were more important, [16.161–165] 'putting him in the end bed rather than in the middle, having things he liked on the bed, a Toy Story video, things he can relate to that make him feel more at home'.

Mum was worried about him running off and getting lost, and about how hospital staff might not understand him. [16.40] 'They are about people being sick, but put it together with a learning disability and I feel, because they are trained on other things, they don't really understand', and [16.43] 'I think it should be a general thing across the board that all people/staff are trained (about learning disability)'.

Communication was a significant issue. Hospital staff showed good insight into how to communicate with someone who has no verbal communication. [15.116–118] 'I spoke to him even though he couldn't speak back to me. If he is not happy you will see the sounds he makes and the expression on his face. I held my hand out and he came to me'.

Mum felt that hospital staff had really listened to her. She made an extra comment [16.216] 'Just to say that I was really pleased to be involved with this (research)'.

Hospital staff commented [15.75–80] 'I think the teamwork was excellent. From a nursing point of view I would say we all deserve a pat on the back'.

There was a positive evaluation of the process of health care from everyone involved.

The main findings of the research study

- The answer to the research question is yes; the use of a pre-admission assessment does improve the process of health care for people with learning disabilities accessing secondary health care services.
- The pre-admission assessment:
  1. Identified the specific health needs of the person, and increased awareness and knowledge of hospital staff of the health needs of people with learning disabilities.
  2. Provided the focus for effective, person-centred care planning to take place.
  3. Helped overcome problems relating to communication, behaviour and under/over-protectiveness.
  4. Gave carers more confidence in hospital staff meeting needs of person.
  5. Increased confidence of hospital staff in working with people with learning disabilities, through feeling better informed and prepared.
  6. Provided a system for joint working to take place, which reduced anxiety for all stake-holders.
  7. Enabled community nurses to act as effective health facilitators, and offer appropriate support to other stakeholders.

Hannon (2003) used a case dynamics matrix (Miles and Hubermann 1994, p. 148) to summarise the pre-admission assessment and its influence on the health care process which is presented in Table 2.1.

Reflective Learning Point:

What are the key points to consider when undertaking a pre-admission assessment of a person with a learning disability?

CARE PLANNING AND DEVELOPING CARE PATHWAYS

Care planning is the process of developing and agreeing an approach to how care is going to be provided for an individual. It is based on meeting the identified individual health care needs, and outlines the roles and responsibilities of people involved in the health care process. Care planning should enable consistent approaches in health care interventions based on best practice guidance. (*See Chapter 1 for further information about person-centred approaches to care planning.*)

HFT (2009) suggests a number of steps that will help hospitals to prepare in advance for the admission of a person with a learning disability including:

- Develop clear policies
- Have identified 'leads' to support people with a learning disability
- Produce easy-to-understand information about the hospital and about different procedures
- Gather resources that can help when a person with a learning disability is admitted
- Provide training to hospital staff on learning disability/disability awareness issues
- Use standard pre-admission assessment tools to assess and identify specific needs

Table 2.1 Case dynamics matrix

Problems identified in the evidence base	Underlying themes	How pre-admission assessment helped
Communication	• Service user needs • Lack of confidence • Lack of training	• Informed and prepared hospital staff • Explained how to communicate • Explained level of comprehension
Behaviour	• Service user needs • Lack of confidence • Lack of training	• Informed and prepared hospital staff • Described behaviours • Informed staff how to respond
Negative attitude of hospital staff	• Limited experience • Disability awareness • Lack of training	• Learning disability nurses able to present a more positive image of person • Prepared hospital staff • Facilitated successful admission leading to positive outcomes
Lack of confidence of hospital staff	• Limited experience • Disability awareness • Lack of training	• Better informed → better prepared → more confident • Active liaison and support from learning disability nurse
Carers need to provide basic care	• Resource implications • Planning • Hospital staff uncertainty and lack of confidence	• Level of support needed clearly identified • Learning disability nurse provided support for carer and hospital staff • Carers more confident in hospital staff meeting needs of service users
Hospital staff not understanding specific needs	• Limited experience • Disability awareness • Lack of training	• Provided detailed, specific information, and enabled person-centred care plan to be developed • Service user consulted • Learning disability nurse acted as health facilitator
Tendency for under/over-protectiveness	• Hospital staff uncertainty of service user needs • Disability awareness • Lack of training	• Identified skill level, areas of competence, and areas where help is needed

- Ensure staff are up to date with the Mental Capacity Act and guidance around 'consent'
- Arrange funding systems to pay for additional support when needed

Bollands and Jones (2002) explained how a review of acute services for people with learning disabilities in Sheffield identified not only the need for more tailored services, but also the need for improved training and more comprehensive patient documentation.

Not all people with a learning disability will have additional needs and many will be able to manage their own health care. This may even include people who have additional support. It is important that during the assessment process the appropriate level of support is identified. For some individuals the fact that they are supported can reduce the interaction that the health care professional has with them.

As a fundamental right to confidentiality, care should be taken to ensure that if the person has the capacity to decide if their carer remains with them during the consultation, this opportunity must be given. This is especially important during any investigation that may be of a personal or intimate nature. From experience the authors have found that people with a learning disability usually want their carer to stay, at least to give emotional support. In some situations, however, the carer attending may be an agency worker who the person does not know well and may feel uncomfortable with their presence during the assessment process.

People with learning disabilities often state their annoyance that an assumption is made that they cannot speak for themselves.

'People (in health services) think that because we have a disability they don't need to talk to us and they talk to our carer instead. This isn't fair, we're people too'. (Joint Committee on Human Rights (2007–8–8))

It is therefore important that decisions about how much support the person needs and wants is assessed as a matter of priority during the pre-admission process. Hannon (2003) found that many people with a learning disability demonstrate a good understanding of their health needs, reason for admission and treatment received.

Reflective Learning Point:

Consider how you would explain a typical health care procedure that you provide to a person with a learning disability.

The role of carers should not go unacknowledged. Many carers express their concerns at the lack of importance put upon the information and support they can offer. Families and carers often report that they feel that medical staff do not listen to them or that their concerns are ignored.

'Many health professionals do not properly consult and involve the families and carers of people with a learning disability'. Mencap (2007)

It may seem that trying to do the right thing by the patient and the carer may cause one or the other to feel that their needs are not being acknowledged. The principle that the individual has capacity to make decisions for themselves unless there is evidence to the contrary (Mental Capacity Act 2004) must be the starting point in any assessment of support need.

Some people may have brought information with them to help you with this. Prior to admission assessment documents, grab sheets and communication passports are becoming more commonly used by learning disability support services and include valuable information for health care providers.

If a person with learning disabilities is admitted unaccompanied, and either requests support or is having difficulties with their assessment or treatment, the triage nurse should attempt to identify a main carer or relative and make contact with them as soon as possible, to assist with the care planning process.

HFT (2009) highlights that 'It is important to note that it is the hospitals' responsibility to fund any extra support over and above any funded support ordinarily available to the person when in their own home'.

Health action plans

An HAP is a personal plan that documents the health needs of an individual. All people with a learning disability are to be offered HAP as part of the Department of Health directive *Valuing People*: A New Strategy for Learning Disability for the Twenty-First Century (Department of Health 2001).

An HAP is usually devised alongside a health screening process completed in the primary health care setting. The HAP documents the health needs of the person with a learning disability and outlines the plan to manage those health needs. This will include any support the person needs to improve and maintain good health.

The HAP must support independence, choice and inclusion. For some individuals a health facilitator may be required to achieve this. The health facilitator is an individual such as a family member, carer or close friend who helps the person with a learning disability with issues related to their health.

Most HAPs are devised with the help of the local learning disability nursing team in conjunction with the patients' GP surgery.

For advice and support regarding health action planning, you should contact your local Learning Disability Service or access the valuing people website: http://valuingpeople.gov.uk/.

Reflective Learning Point:

Why is it important to involve family/carers in care planning?

Developing care pathways

The development of local care pathways/protocols offers a framework for individual person-centred planning to take place, reducing variation in practice, and improving care provided. It also provides higher levels of consistency in approach and standards of care.

Using a simple framework and agreeing care pathways in advance can help to highlight and overcome any issues that may arise, and to alleviate any concerns of the person with a learning disability, their family/carers and health professionals involved in the health care process.

Figure 2.6 outlines a simple template for a care pathway for people with a learning disability who require dental treatment under general anaesthetic. It incorporates person-centred assessment and care planning based on identified needs, best practice guidance on obtaining consent, and a simple process that clearly outlines who does what in the process of health care. You could use this template as a basic model to add to, or also adapt it to other scenarios.

INTERVENTION AND TREATMENT

The basis to all interventions and treatment is communication; giving people an explanation of what is going to happen to them and why you are doing this. Developing a relationship with the person, getting to know them and interacting with them prior to undertaking any interventions can help to ensure successful outcomes. It is important to ensure the person and their carers are given a full explanation of procedures and to check that they have understood this, giving them the opportunity to ask questions if they wish.

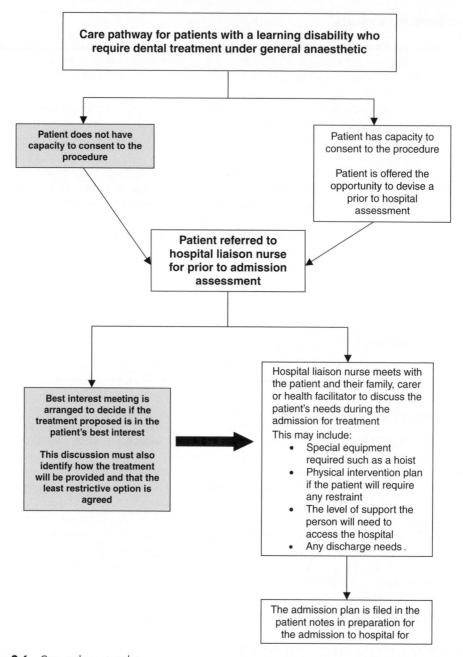

Fig. 2.6 Care pathway template.

For those patients with learning disability where communication is difficult, you may need to use alternative means of communications such as sign language, symbols, photographs or objects of reference. (*See Chapter 3 for further information on methods and tools for communication.*)

A very common concern for families and carers using general hospital services is the amount of time spent waiting in busy, noisy waiting areas. Hannon (2003) reported that 'people felt it was generally better to get treatment early in the day rather than waiting', and you may consider this when planning your intervention and treatment.

It is acknowledged that hospital services are busy places with triage systems that prioritise patient need, and that it can be very distressing for all patients who are experiencing pain and discomfort to have to wait their turn. However, most patients are able to identify the constraints of the department and may express their displeasure but on the whole are able to manage themselves during this time. For carers of people with a learning disability this level of discomfort can be magnified by the challenge of supporting someone who is injured or unwell, who is unable to comprehend what is going to happen to them, and is in an unfamiliar environment with minimal support.

Emergency Triage (Manchester Triage Group 1997) acknowledges that 'Apart from extremes of age, there will be patients who have particular difficulties. These include those with special needs, poor eye sight, poor hearing etc. People who can cope quite well in the community under controlled circumstances may have great difficulties in the strange environment of the emergency department. Communication again becomes particularly important, and it may be appropriate for such patients to be seen quite quickly'.

The National Patient Safety Agency (NPSA; 2004) reports that anxiety about waiting times is a common concern for people with learning disabilities and their family or carers, especially those with complex needs. The time spent waiting often causes the person to become more anxious and therefore their ability to focus on the consultation and answer questions or be able to tolerate tests or investigations is very much affected. Making the appointment at the start of the list is an obvious solution to ensure that the person is seen as near to the appointment time as possible.

It is also important for the health care professional leading the clinic to be aware of any problems occurring in the waiting area and to respond as quickly as possible when the patient needs to be seen as soon as possible, which may require them being seen before another patient. From our experience of sitting with an anxious patient, other patients waiting are very supportive and are more concerned for the person's anxiety than missing their turn.

Carers will provide valuable feedback on how the person responds to your interventions and any changes to their condition. HFT (2009, p. 13) suggests 'including family carers and/or paid support staff in the nursing handover, or at least seek information from them to share at the handover'. They will also offer good support for changing needs, for example explaining when it will be appropriate to leave a person unaccompanied in hospital during their treatment, and when they will need someone with them.

Reflective Learning Point:

How would you make 'reasonable adjustments' in your department for a person with a learning disability attending for a treatment intervention?

A2A is a national group of health care professionals from both hospital and learning disability services who work together to identify and suggest ways to overcome barriers to health care for people with a learning disability. The following information is reproduced (with permission) from one of their documents:

Disabling practice – and how to avoid it
Providing equal access for disabled patients in the NHS
A disabled patient is first and foremost a patient
Do not make assumptions
This is some simple guidance which we hope will help you to work better with disabled people with a range of needs.

Talking
- Relax – disabled people are used to other people saying inappropriate things
- Try to avoid labels
- Avoid jargon – use simple language and speak clearly
- Talk to the disabled person and not their carer
- Do not speak too fast – many people with a learning disability have a hearing impairment

Listening
- Do not be afraid to ask a patient to repeat if you do not hear what they say
- Ask about how best to listen and communicate – sometimes pen and paper can help – if it is the patient's choice
- Ask for clarification if needed
- Use 'objects of reference' for non-verbal communication

Facilitating
- Consider rearranging the room or using a different room with easier access
- Have different types of seating available, for example high back chair, chair with arms
- Provide information in different formats, for example larger print, pictures
- Extra time might be needed for some people
- Ask the person what help they need and respect their answer
- Involve carers (with consent) in the discussions

Supporting
- Provide written information in advance to allow people time to find out about what is going to happen
- Give clear directions and information
- Be positive towards the patient – only discuss disability issues when relevant for their treatment
- Ensure all information is in a useable and accessible format
- Consider the involvement of other professionals who can help – LD nurse, speech and language therapist, PALS etc.

(See Chapter 3 for detailed information about communication matters.)

Practical support in hospital

The National Patient Safety Agency (2004) identified four key areas where hospital staff can provide practical support for people with learning disabilities while they are patients in hospital:

1. *Food*: Some people found it difficult to choose their meal because the menu option was not in an accessible format. For others there is an inability to feed themselves due to a variety of reasons, from being physically unable to hold the cutlery to not understanding that the tray at the end of the bed is their food for them to eat.

As part of the pre-admission assessment those patients who are unable to read must be asked if they would like to receive support to complete their menu and how they would like this support to be given. The level of support each person needs for food must be clearly identified and outlined in their notes.

2. *Access*: The access issues noted by NPSA were not only about the lack of ramps and signs. For one person not being able to reach the call button to ask for help, because it was behind her head where she could not reach, prevented her from getting to the toilet in time. Fortunately, she had not needed to call for help due to a medical emergency.

It is important when relying on the patient to alert the health care professional when they require assistance that the person understands how to use the call system and that the call system is accessible for the person to use. For many people with learning disabilities the call button is not a suitable system and therefore a suitable replacement must be identified. In most cases it is more appropriate that a health care professional be allocated to monitor the patient during each shift to identify when the patient needs assistance.

3. *Staff responses to patients with learning difficulties*: Some people with a learning disability report they feel they do not receive the physical support they need. Most commonly this is with reference to eating and drinking. It is important to establish the level of physical support the person needs during their admission to hospital. For some this may be very different from the level of support they may have needed in their own home. The pre-admission assessment process described earlier in this chapter can ensure that all aspects of personal care support can be identified and the relevant support needs documented.

4. *Link between community learning difficulty services and hospital*: The pre-admission assessment can provide essential information to ensure that hospital services are aware of how best to support a person with learning disabilities. NPSA also recommends link workers in hospitals to support both the patient and the health care professionals.

The Royal College of Nursing (RCN; 2006, p. 11) outlined a number of suggestions of how health care professionals can support people with a learning disability to access hospital services including:

- *Preparation*:
  - Find out about the person's communication abilities
  - Talk to people who know them
  - Think about the words you use when talking to people
  - Offer first appointments and longer appointments
  - Consider offering a home visit
  - Give information beforehand
- *Environment*:
  - Make sure lighting is not too bright
  - Avoid any sudden noise
  - Avoid too much clutter
  - Ensure environment is physically accessible for the person
- *Verbal and written communication*:
  - Always speak to the person with a learning disability first, not the person supporting them
  - Speak clearly and not too fast
  - Check the person understands what you have said
  - Use symbols and photographs if appropriate

Mencap (2004, p. 23) also made a number of recommendations for key actions that could improve the health and the experience of the heath care process for people with a learning disability:

(a) Better training in learning disability for all health care staff
(b) Longer and more flexible appointments
(c) Accessible information to be provided in all health care settings
(d) All screening programmes to ensure that people with a learning disability have the same access rate as others
(e) Identification on health records that someone has a learning disability
(f) Tackle health inequalities through the health equity audit
(g) Annual health checks offered to all people with a learning disability (with GP)
(h) Hospitals to fulfil legal duty of care and provide appropriate levels of support to patients with a learning disability
(i) An inquiry into premature deaths

Actions have already been taken at both a policy and practical levels in response to these recommendations in both primary and secondary health care services. As outlined previously, it is often simple adjustments with consideration of individual needs that has the greatest benefit.

Reflective Learning Point:

What kind of practical support can help a person with a learning disability during their stay in hospital?

Prescribing and taking medication

The National Patient Safety Agency (2004) noted particular concerns that people were unclear about the medication they were prescribed. It was identified that people often associate their medication by its shape and/or colour.

For some people, changes of the type of medication without the thought of any difficulties the person may have taking it was an issue. Some people who, for whatever reason, have difficulty swallowing their medication were found to have their medication withheld for long periods of time until an alternative medication or method of administration is decided by the doctor. This can have potentially serious implications for individuals, for example especially those whose epilepsy is controlled by a strict time regulated regime.

The NPSA recommend that information regarding the medication and its administration should be provided in a format that is accessible to the person. This may include using bigger labels on the bottles and using language or symbols more appropriate for the persons' needs as illustrated in Figure 2.7.

For some individuals the change in their medication regime can be confusing and the person is at high risk of potential discrepancies in the way they take their medication on discharge. Wherever possible the person should be monitored self-administrating prior to discharge to ensure that they are fully conversant with the medication they are prescribed, and how and when

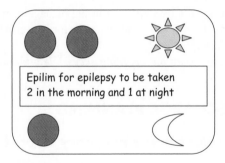

Fig. 2.7   Example of an accessible label.

it should be taken. If it is evident that the person is not competent in the management of their medication alternatives need to be established.

Below is an example of a medication sheet for Mary. The shape and colour of the tablets are an accurate representation of each tablet. Mary places each tablet on the sheet to ensure she takes the correct tablet at the right time (Fig. 2.8).

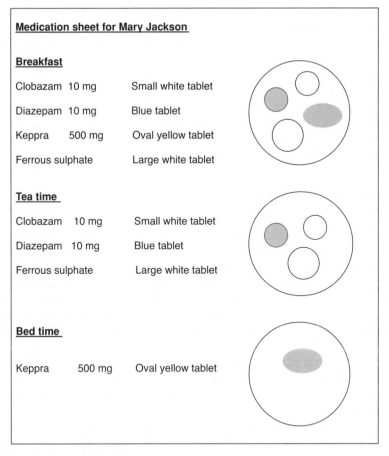

Fig. 2.8   Example of a medication sheet.

Accessible information is not only important in the management of safe medicine administration, but NPSA also highlights the need for *all* information provided for patients to be provided in an accessible format.

(See Chapter 3 for more information regarding accessible information.)

LIAISON AND DISCHARGE PLANNING

Discharge from accident and emergency department

When discharging a person with a learning disability from the emergency department, it is important that the named nurse assesses what follow-up is required and makes any necessary referrals to other agencies. This may be due to concerns such as the patient's safety, mental health and/or challenging behaviour, the patient's ability to comprehend instructions regarding follow-up care or follow medication regimens.

Some patients may have a personal health record that they may ask you to complete with them. This document is commonly known in learning disability services as an HAP (see earlier notes) and is used as a communication tool for the person with a learning disability to ensure that all those involved in providing care and support have information to help the person maintain a healthy lifestyle. A brief summary of the treatment received and any follow-up appointments or prescribed medication should be documented.

Care should be given if providing leaflets explaining discharge care to clarify if the patient is able to read. It is recommended that all departments provide information in accessible formats (with pictures and diagrams) to aid understanding. Your local learning disability service would be able to help you with this.

Health care professionals in general hospitals should consider contacting social services, mental health services, the community learning disability team or, if your hospital has one, the LD liaison nurse. These services would be able to follow up the patient at home to establish if they are following discharge advice and provide any further support required.

General liaison and discharge planning

Due to the possible complexities of preparing for discharge of a person with a learning disability, discussion regarding discharge should be raised with the person and their main carer at the time of admission. Where cases are particularly complex you may also want to involve the acute liaison nurse, social services and the community learning disabilities team in the planning.

The Department of Health (2003) identifies key principles for effective discharge and transfer of care which recommends a whole system's approach to discharge planning that ensures active participation of individuals and their carers and that discharge is not an isolated event and should be coordinated from pre-admission planning right through discharge. Hospital discharge legislation and guidance will generally also advise that carers must be involved in discharge planning. Professor Nigel Sparrows (Royal College of General Practitioners 2009) identifies that to make an effective diagnosis, accurate information is required, and it is often the carer which provides a vital link between patient and doctor. He adds that it is important that carers feel supported and valued in this role.

There may be a variety of issues that can significantly affect the success of discharge for people with learning disabilities, the main issue being the changes that may be required to the level of care they currently have commissioned.

Process of Health Care Case Study 6 – Discharge Planning

Michael is 67 and was admitted to hospital after a fall at home. He did not sustain any injuries but it was identified that he had developed diabetes and the fall was probably due to his blood sugar level. Michael is much better but he is struggling with his mobility. It is felt that this is probably due to him lacking confidence after his fall. However, he is medically fit for discharge and the ward has called his home to say he is ready to leave. Unfortunately, the ward has not considered that Michael lives in a terraced house with two other men and his bedroom is upstairs. The staff are not available to attend to Michael at night if he needs support and are concerned about him returning home with his current level of mobility.

This case study highlights that people with learning disabilities live in a variety of housing situations. The majority will live in their own home, either alone or with family or carers. Some people will receive part-time support, and others will receive a full package of care that supports them 24 hours a day, but this may be shared care and does not necessarily mean that they will have one-to-one care throughout the day and night. It is therefore important to establish with carers the level of support provided and identify any circumstances that may delay discharge, either until the person is recovered more fully and is able to be safely discharged home, or if additional support or change of accommodation is required.

It is unfortunate that due to the pressures of discharging, some people with learning disabilities are forced to be transferred to other environments. This is often just for a couple of days, until they are sufficiently recovered to return home, but this can often be confusing and distressing for the individual. The Department of Health (2003) advises the development of protocols to establish access to specialist advice for people with learning disabilities and that the ward should liaise with the health or social care professional supporting the individual to ensure effective discharge planning.

A discharge planning meeting should take place with all relevant parties to think about and identify what the person will need when they leave the hospital. This may include changes to living arrangements, equipment or additional support that they do not usually receive.

HFT (2009) suggests the following steps for hospitals to follow when it is time for the person with a learning disability to leave hospital:

- Organise a formal discharge meeting
- Inform family/carers/support staff of any requirements following the hospital stay, such as side effects of new medication or what to do if any complications arise
- Check arrangements for any outstanding specialist assessments, for example occupational therapy
- Inform the community learning disability team that the person is leaving hospital
- Organise transport if needed
- Invite the person, their family/carers and support staff to give feedback on the hospital experience – what has gone well and what could be improved

As discussed previously the person may have an HAP. This should be reviewed prior to discharge and any necessary additions or amendments should be made with the relevant person informed of these changes to the HAP. If the person does not have an HAP this may be an appropriate time to initiate one and advice regarding this can be obtained from the acute liaison nurse or local learning disability team.

If the person is to be discharged with medication the discharging nurse must ensure that the person is able to administer their medication independently. If there are concerns that the patient may have difficulties taking their medication as prescribed, pharmacy services may be able to help or the acute liaison nurse will be able to provide follow-up support.

On the day of discharge a copy of the discharge plan, detailing care needs on discharge, should be given to the main carer and a copy sent to the community learning disabilities team if they are involved. The GP should be notified and the district nursing service should be contacted for any standard community nurse follow-up, for example removal of sutures, dressings etc. Feedback from all stakeholders involved during the admission and discharge will enable learning to take place, promote service development, improve standards and enhance the process of care for the future.

Reflective Learning Point:

What information would you need to know when planning the discharge of a person with a learning disability?

CONCLUSION

This chapter set out to explore the process of health care for people with a learning disability accessing general hospital services, and highlights the key stages in the patient journey, from assessment and admission through successful interventions and discharge.

The importance and benefits of a detailed pre-admission assessment are outlined, and a number of flowcharts are provided to aid care planning through different aspects of general hospital services.

When working with people with a learning disability, it is important for health care professionals to consider some of the important factors that influence the health care process, and use a person-centred care planning process to overcome any barriers to health care and provide the practical support that each individual may need during their stay.

Summary of Key Learning Points

The key learning points are:

- Pre-admission assessment and person-centred care planning is the key to a successful admission.
- Developing care pathways within departments can make things easier.
- Allowing sufficient time is a significant factor that influences the health care process. This may be time to spend with the individual or time for explanations.
- An introductory visit is useful for some people.
- Flexibility in appointment systems, offering first or longer appointments can help some people.
- Prepare information about the hospital and different procedures in easy-to-understand formats.

- Develop communication systems and resources for use to explain interventions to the individual.
- Disability awareness training for the staff team can help influence attitudes and aid understanding of needs.
- Liaison and joint working with the person, their family/carer and other professionals helps to ensure successful interventions.

Links to Key KSF Competencies – Chapter 2

	Level descriptors			
Core dimensions	**1**	**2**	**3**	**4**
1 – Communication	Communicate with a limited range of people on day-to-day matters	Communicate with a range of people on a range of matters	Develop and maintain communication with people about difficult matters and/or in difficult situations	Develop and maintain communication with people on complex matters, issues and ideas and/or in complex situations
2 – Personal and people development	Contribute to own personal development	Develop own skills and knowledge and provide information to others to help their development	Develop oneself and contribute to the development of others	Develop oneself and others in areas of practice
3 – Health safety and security	Assist in maintaining own and others' health, safety and security	Monitor and maintain health, safety and security of self and others	Promote, monitor and maintain best practice in health, safety and security	Maintain and develop an environment and a culture that improves health, safety and security
4 – Service improvement	Make changes in own practice and offer suggestions for improving services	Contribute to the improvement of services	Appraise, interpret and apply suggestions, recommendations and directives to improve services	Work in partnership with others to develop, take forward and evaluate direction, policies and strategies
5 – Quality	Maintain the quality of own work	Maintain quality in own work and encourage others to do so	Contribute to improving quality	Develop a culture that improves quality
6 – Equality and diversity	Act in ways that support equality and value diversity	Support equality and value diversity	Promote equality and value diversity	Develop a culture that promotes equality and values diversity

Health and well-being	Level descriptors			
	1	**2**	**3**	**4**
HWB1 – Promotion of health and well-being and prevention of adverse effects on health and well-being	Contribute to promoting health and well-being and preventing adverse effects on health and well-being	Plan, develop and implement approaches to promote health and well-being and prevent adverse effects on health and well-being	Plan, develop and implement programmes to promote health and well-being and prevent adverse effects on health and well-being	Promote health and well-being and prevent adverse effects on health and well-being through contributing to the development, implementation and evaluation of related policies
HWB2 – Assessment and care planning to meet health and well-being needs	Assist in the assessment of people's health and well-being needs	Contribute to assessing health and well-being needs and planning how to meet those needs	Assess health and well-being needs and develop, monitor and review care plans to meet specific needs	Assess complex health and well-being needs and develop, monitor and review care plans to meet those needs
HWB3 – Protection of health and well-being	Recognise and report situations where there might be a need for protection	Contribute to protecting people at risk	Implement aspects of a protection plan and review its effectiveness	Develop and lead on the implementation of an overall protection plan
HWB4 – Enablement to address health and well-being needs	Help people meet daily health and well-being needs	Enable people to meet ongoing health and well-being needs	Enable people to address specific needs in relation to health and well-being	Empower people to realise and maintain their potential in relation to health and well-being
HWB5 – Provision of care to meet health and well-being needs	Undertake care activities to meet individuals' health and well-being needs	Undertake care activities to meet the health and well-being needs of individuals with a greater degree of dependency	Plan, deliver and evaluate care to meet people's health and well-being needs	Plan, deliver and evaluate care to address people's complex health and well-being needs
HWB6 – Assessment and treatment planning	Undertake tasks related to the assessment of physiological and psychological functioning	Contribute to the assessment of physiological and psychological functioning	Assess physiological and psychological functioning and develop, monitor and review related treatment plans	Assess physiological and psychological functioning when there are complex and/or undifferentiated abnormalities, diseases and disorders and develop, monitor and review related treatment plans

HWB7 – Interventions and treatments	Assist in providing interventions and/or treatments	Contribute to planning, delivering and monitoring interventions and/or treatments	Plan, deliver and evaluate interventions and/or treatments	Plan, deliver and evaluate interventions and/or treatments when there are complex issues and/or serious illness

Department of Health (2004). Reproduced under the terms of the Click-Use Licence.

REFERENCES

A2A – Access to Acute: A network for staff working with people with learning disabilities to support access to acute medical treatment (2009). Available at http://www.nnldn.org.uk/a2a/. Contact: rick.robson@sssft.nhs.uk.

Bollands R and Jones A (2002) Improving care for people with learning disabilities. *Nursing Times*, 98(35), 38–39.

Brown M (2005) Emergency care for people with learning disabilities: what all nurses and midwives need to know. *Accident and Emergency Nursing*, 13(4), 224–231.

Brown M and MacArthur J (1999) Discrimination on grounds of need not disabilities. *Nursing Times*, 95, 29.

Cooper S A, Melville C and Morrison J (2004) People with intellectual disabilities: their health needs differ and need to be recognised and met. *British Medical Journal*, 239, 414–415.

Davis D and Evans L (2001) Assessing pain in people with profound learning disabilities. *British Journal of Nursing*, 10(8), 513–516.

Davis S and Marsden R (2001) Disabled people in hospital: evaluating the clinical nurse specialist (CNS) role. *Nursing Standard*, 15(21), 33–37.

Disability Discrimination Act (1995) HMSO, London.

Department of Health (2001) *Valuing People*. HMSO, London.

Department of Health (2003) *Discharge from Hospital: Pathway, Process and Practice*. HMSO, London. www.doh.gov.uk/jointunit.

Department of Health (2004) *The NHS Knowledge and Skills Framework (NHS KSF) and the Development Review Process. Appendix 1: Overview of the NHS KSF*. HMSO, London.

Department of Health (2005) *Mental Capacity Act*. HMSO, London.

Department of Health (2008) *Carers at the Heart of 21st Century Families and Communities*. HMSO, London.

Hannon L (2003) *Pre-Admission Assessment in Secondary Healthcare Services for People with Learning Disabilities*. Unpublished MSc Dissertation. University of Central Lancashire, UK.

HFT (2009) *Working Together: Easy Steps to Improving How People with a Learning Disability Are Supported When in Hospital (Guidance for Hospitals, Families and Paid Support Staff)*. HFT, Gloucester, UK.

House of Lords, House of Commons, Joint Committee on Human Rights (2007–2008) *A Life Like Any Other? Human Rights of Adults with Learning Disabilities*. The House of Commons. London: The Stationary Office.

Manchester Triage Group (1997) *Emergency Triage*. BMJ Publishing Group, London.

Mencap (1998) *Health for All*. Mencap, London.

Mencap (2004) *Treat Me Right! Better Healthcare for People with a Learning Disability*. Mencap, London.

Mencap (2007) *Death by Indifference*. Mencap, London.

Miles M and Hubermann A (1994) *Qualitative Data Analysis*. Sage, London.

Morgan (2000) cited in Brown M (2005) Emergency care for people with learning disabilities: what all nurses and midwives need to know. *Accident and Emergency Nursing*, 13(4), 224–231.

National Patient Safety Agency (2004) *Listening to People with Learning Difficulties and Family Carers Talk about Patient Safety*. NPSA, London.

Øvretveit J (1998) *Evaluating Health Interventions*. Open University Press, Buckingham.

Ploeg J (1999) Identifying the best research design to fit the question. Part 2. Qualitative designs. *Evidence-Based Nursing*, 2(2), 36–37.

Ritchie J and Spencer L (1993) In: Bryman A and Burgess R (eds). *Analysing Qualitative Data*. Routledge, London.

Royal College of General Practitioners (2009) Supporting carers: an action guide for general practitioners and their team. Available at www.rcgp.org.uk.

Royal College of Nursing (RCN) (2002) *Defining Nursing*. RCN, London.

Royal College of Nursing (RCN) (2006) *Meeting the Health Needs of People with Learning Disabilities: Guidance for Nursing Staff*. RCN, London.

3 Communication

INTRODUCTION

The evidence base highlights communication as one of the most significant issues for people with a learning disability admitted to hospital. This chapter explores the key issues related to communicating with people with a learning disability and identifies the important skills that health care professionals working in general hospitals need to enable effective communication to take place. Guidance is provided on how to identify if someone has communication difficulties and a range of ideas presented for how to overcome these and respond appropriately to people's communication needs. Examples of tools to aid communication are included, with information about how advocacy and empowerment can be used to help people with a learning disability to make choices.

An estimated 26% of people with a learning disability are admitted to hospital each year compared with 14% of the general population (NHS Health Scotland 2004). Of those people, it is estimated that around 40% will have moderate or severe hearing impairment, 50% will have significant communication difficulties and around 80% of people with learning disabilities have some level of communication problem.

As outlined in Chapter 2, the basis to all health care interventions and treatment is communication, giving people an explanation of what is going to happen to them and why you are doing this. Developing a relationship with the person, getting to know them and interacting with them prior to undertaking any interventions can help to ensure successful outcomes. It is important to ensure the person and their carers are given a full explanation of procedures and to check that they have understood this, giving them the opportunity to ask questions if they wish.

The Royal College of Nursing (2006, p. 11) highlights that 'Accessible information and good communication skills are crucial if people with learning disabilities are to have equal access to primary and secondary health care. People need to be able to access information they can understand and with which they can make decisions about their health. People with learning disabilities also need information on how to stay well'. They recommend that all health care settings should have a summary of key points on:

- How to communicate with people with learning disabilities
- How to write accessible information
- Duties under the Disability Discrimination Act (DDA) (Department of Health 1995) to treat all patients equally, whenever reasonably possible, irrespective of their disability

General Hospital Care for People with Learning Disabilities, First Edition by Lynn Hannon and Julie Clift
© 2011 Blackwell Publishing Ltd

For those patients with a learning disability where communication is difficult, you may need to use alternative means of communications such as sign language, symbols, photographs or objects of reference, which are all discussed within this chapter.

WHAT IS COMMUNICATION?

There are many definitions of communication that generally cover the fact that it is a way of giving and receiving information, or imparting knowledge, that involves verbal or written contact with another.

Abudarham and Hurd (2002, p. 193) quote Light (1997), who states that 'Communication is the essence of human life', and that (Light 1988) 'Communication is the means by which the individual can express needs and wants, develop social closeness, exchange information and fulfil social etiquette routines'. They suggest that 'it should be considered as a human right, and an opportunity that should be available to all individuals equally, in order that they can develop socially, emotionally and cognitively'. They continue to recommend that 'It is the responsibility of carers and professionals in that person's environment to ensure that an individual who is unable to communicate effectively by oral means has a means of communicating that can be interpreted by others'.

Cogher (2005) summarises the critical features of communication as:

- It is at least two way
- It may be verbal or non-verbal
- It may not always be successful
- Interpretation is needed

Cogher highlights that for communication to be effective those who are in the communication relationship need to have a shared social and cultural link. Communication ability is dependent on our opportunities and experience of the world, from how we were raised, and in what part of the world we developed our communication skills. We all have very different communication ability. Some of us will have had experiences that have allowed the acquisition of a foreign language, or will have studied at university and developed a vocabulary particular to the area of study.

However, no matter how well developed our communication skills are, there will be times when we misunderstand what someone is trying to communicate to us. The two-way process of communication can be affected by the person's ability to express themselves, and the ability of the person receiving the message to hear and understand what is being said.

Reflective Learning point:

Those of you living in Lancashire will understand what is being asked if someone says to you, 'do you want a brew?' If you have experience of living in Lancashire, or have contact with someone there, you will know that you are being asked if you would like a cup of tea. In the West Midlands you might say that the cup of tea is 'bostin' which suggests that you think your cup of tea is really good.

Think about what expressions you use every day in health care that may not be understood by the patient?

Perception and comprehension

Perception is the process we use to collect, interpret and comprehend information from the world around us by means of our senses. The first stage in our development of perception is by taking in the sensations and experiencing them without attaching any meaning to them. With gradual development and maturation we begin to interpret the sensations and develop a comprehension of the incoming information.

Stimulus → Sensation → Interpretation → Comprehension

Some people with learning disabilities, especially those with autism, have particular difficulty with perception and abstract understanding, leading to difficulties with interpretation and comprehension. They have a literal understanding of what you say.

Many people with a mild learning disability may have problems with understanding idioms and inferences. They may also have difficulties with understanding some of these higher level language functions. Some people with learning disabilities have problems understanding complex issues, for example the choice of treatment, particularly if they are upset or anxious (Fig. 3.1).

You may have seen the illusion known as the 'Kanizsa triangle' before. Bogdashina (2005) explains that 'Non-autistic individuals report they *see* a triangle. But the triangle does not exist. It is our mind that makes the blank space meaningful'. She continues 'Those autistic individuals who have acquired certain conceptual knowledge also succumb to these illusions . . . while those who are at the stage of literal perception do not see the triangle'.

How we experience and interpret the world around us is dependant on our memories and experience. What a person perceives often reflects past experience, and present beliefs and states of mind. Bogdashina (2005) gives this example, 'a Conservative and Labour MP who listen to the same speech will "hear" different things and will make different conclusions'. Therefore,

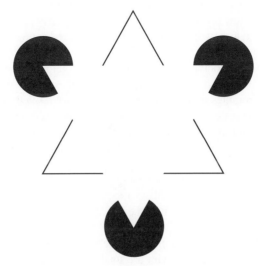

Fig. 3.1   The Kanizsa triangle.

it is important to acknowledge that we do not perceive the things we see and hear in the same way, nor will we make the same conclusions from the message communicated to us.

Communication Case Study 1 – (Comprehension) – David

David has difficulties understanding verbal information. He can understand only one word in a sentence. He needs to use the cues of the routine and non-verbal cues to understand what is going to happen. David needs a blood test. He has been prepared by his carer and knows that he is to have a blood test; however, David appears anxious and repeats, 'hurt no'.

David sits in the chair with the nurse. The nurse tells David 'I'm going to take some blood now David, it won't hurt if you stay nice and still and then you can go home'. David gets up from the chair and goes to the door.

It is possible that David took his understanding from two parts of this statement that influenced his action,

1. 'hurt' – David may not want the blood test if it is going to hurt and so decides to get up and leave.
2. 'go home' – David may understand that it is time to go home.

Although this statement is typical in a situation like this and is made with all good intention to reassure and support the patient it did not have the result intended. The nurse may have had a more successful outcome if she had limited her verbal interaction.

- The nurse could give gentle reassurance by her body language, by sitting near David and when he says 'hurt, no' the nurse could repeat 'no'.
- The nurse could give a cue by touching his arm and saying 'stay here'.
- The nurse should then proceed with taking the blood saying 'blood test now'.

By minimising the verbal interaction and giving support by gestures and gentle body language, this will minimise any misunderstanding on the part of the patient.

Abstract concepts such as how the person understands time are often problematic in a health care situation. For some people who have difficulty with these concepts being told 'you will be going to theatre later' or 'the doctor will be coming to see you tomorrow' are meaningless. You will probably find that the person will continue to ask the question even if you have only given them the answer a few minutes before. Patients' anxiety around waiting for appointments or procedures can be minimised by the use of visual aids, written prompts and consistency in the use of language relating to time, for example 'soon'. For people to be able to understand these concepts they need to have the skills to understand time, and this can be enhanced by the use of diaries and calendars.

People who have learning disabilities have a huge range of communication difficulties and each person will have communication needs that vary considerably. For most it is the difficulty with comprehension which can be difficult to accurately assess because as Kelly (2000) explains 'some people with learning disabilities have developed effective social speech and learnt phrases which reap benefits in terms of social contact, but which are sometimes meaningless in terms of content'. Equally, some individuals who are unable to express themselves verbally or by gestures due to conditions such as cerebral palsy may have a good understanding of what is being said to them.

Often people with a learning disability are thought to be having problems with their memory or are developing dementia when it is really a matter of comprehension. Most people with a learning disability will have some level of difficulty with language comprehension. It can often be unclear how much the patient who has a learning disability understands of what you are asking or information you need to relay to them regarding their treatment and care. We are often reliant on carers or family members to give guidance on how to communicate with someone, or to establish how much they will understand.

A common response may be 'oh they understand everything you say to them', but you should always clarify the level of comprehension for each intervention as this may change. Clake, Kehoe and Harris (1992), in Kevan (2003), demonstrated that there is often a mismatch between what staff believe the person can understand and the client's actual receptive ability. It is always important to check someone has listened and understood what you have said before carrying out any health care intervention.

The following case study illustrates that unfortunately even with the best planning it can be a simple misunderstanding of information that can prevent the success of an intervention.

Communication Case Study 2 – (Comprehension) – Jim

Jim has autism and had been well prepared for his sigmoidoscopy with accessible information in language that he could understand. He also had a preparatory visit to the endoscopy unit. Jim knew that he would be having an enema prior to the procedure and was ready for the enema to be administered. The nurse informed Jim when she was ready to administer the enema that she would be using jelly that may feel a little cold.

This was part of the plan that had been overseen. There had been no explanation of the need for lubricant prior to insertion of the enema. Jim would not let the nurse continue. For Jim 'Jelly' is something you eat and no explanation at this time would convince him that it was OK to use it for this process.

Jim's case highlights the need to be very clear about how the person communicates and the language they use when planning how to best help them understand their treatment. For Jim 'jelly' is something he has at teatime with fruit. If the nurse had stated that she was using a lubricant or gel he may have accepted and agreed to continue. Prior to the next admission this information was added to the accessible information and Jim was shown the lubricant to gain an understanding that the gel is not the same as the jelly he eats at teatime. Jim needed time to be able to process the information that 'lubricating gel' is sometimes known as jelly. Unfortunately for Jim this explanation did not help him and an alternative bowel preparation was needed for the sigmoidoscopy to go ahead. The intervention was then successfully carried out.

Reflective Learning Point:

Joe is a 56-year-old man who has been admitted for surgery. His consent form has been completed during the pre-operative process. On the morning of surgery Joe is sat by his bed in his gown ready to go to theatre and is visited by the surgeon and anaesthetist to establish that Joe is ready to go ahead with his surgery. When Joe is asked what he understands about the procedure he is unable to tell the doctors what he knows.
Is Joe able to consent to this procedure?

The Mental Capacity Act (Department of Health 2005) gives very good guidance regarding how to enhance the communication environment that is relevant in any communication situation but most relevant when it is essential that the person is given every opportunity to express their needs.

It is essential that the person feels at ease. For Joe it is likely that he feels anxious. He is in an unfamiliar environment, there are a number of people around his bed (think about ward rounds when there can be a number of doctors, students and nurses standing around the bed, all looking down on you, how intimidating must that feel?) Joe feels unsure about what to say.

Therefore to ensure that the person is given the best opportunity to communicate their needs, the health care professional should ensure that the environment is appropriate and helps the person to feel at ease and that any decisions are made at a time that is best for the individual. It may also be important to have a familiar person available to support the individual who can help the person to express themselves. (*See Chapter 5 for further information about obtaining consent.*)

MODELS OF COMMUNICATION – VERBAL AND NON-VERBAL

If we define communication as a way of giving or receiving information, effective communication can be measured by how well the information is passed between the two parties. The model in Figure 3.2 illustrates the key components of effective communication.

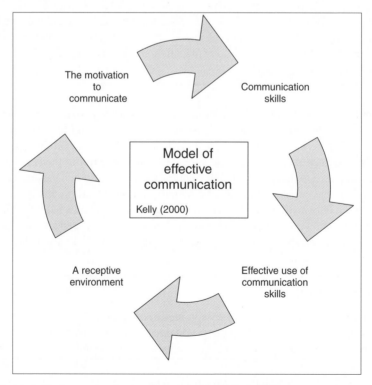

Fig. 3.2   Model of effective communication. Copyright Alex Kelly (2000).

This model suggests that for communication to be effective the communicator must have the desire to communicate with a receiver and have both the skills to communicate and be able to use those skills effectively. The communicator then needs the receiver to be receptive to the communication, which requires the receiver to be both receptive to the communication and to have the ability to understand what the communicator is communicating. For people with learning disabilities this cycle has the potential to be disrupted at each step of the process. (*See later section in this chapter about communicating with people with a learning disability.*)

When exploring models of communication it is helpful to explore the relationship between what we say and what is understood. Mehrabian (1971) suggests that there are three elements to face communication and that the way the message is received by the other person is influenced by:

- 7% of what you say
- 43% intonation in voice
- 55% body language

It is important that health care professionals pay attention to the non-verbal behaviour of both themself and the patient during their interactions. Silverman et al. (2005, p. 123) highlight that 'we need to recognise patient's non-verbal cues in their speech patterns, facial expression, affect and body posture. But we also need to be aware of our own non-verbal behaviour, how the use of eye contact, body position and posture, movement, facial expression and use of voice can all influence the success of the consultation'. They continue to outline (p. 123) the following behaviours or cues that contribute to non-verbal communication, illustrated in Box 3.1.

Mehrabian (1971) states that the non-verbal elements are particularly important for communicating feelings and attitude, especially when they are incongruent: if words and body language disagree, one tends to believe the body language. This would be the case if someone said to you 'How lovely to see you' and at the same time avoids eye contact and has closed body language, you would immediately identify the insincerity of the statement.

In such situations Mehrabian's research showed that the receiver of the communication will accept the predominant form of communication, the non-verbal signals, rather than the literal meaning of the words. Therefore, it is important to be congruent when we communicate. That is, our body language and tone of voice are consistent with the words we use. The words

---

Box 3.1   What do we mean by non-verbal communication?

- *Posture*: sitting, standing, erect, relaxed
- *Proximity*: use of space, physical distance between and positioning of communicators
- *Touch*: handshake, pat, physical contact during examination
- *Body movements*: hand and arm gestures, fidgeting, nodding, foot and leg movements
- *Facial expression*: raised eyebrows, frown, smile, crying
- *Eye behaviour*: eye contact, gaze, staring
- *Vocal cues*: pitch, rate, volume, rhythm, silence, pause, intonation, speech errors
- *Use of time*: early, late, on time, over time, rushed, slow to respond
- *Physical presence*: race, gender, body shape, clothing, grooming
- *Environmental cues*: location, furniture placement, lighting, temperature, colour

Silverman et al. (2005, p. 123). Reproduced with kind permission of Radcliffe Publishing Ltd.

we choose to use are generally more important than is often assumed. This is particularly relevant when spoken language is not the person's main method of communicating their needs. Chambers (2003) describes the use of non-verbal communication skills to improve nursing care. He suggests that in supporting people with severe learning disabilities the main resource is the nurse's 'face, voice and body'.

The non-verbal elements are particularly important in the communication of feelings and attitude. If understanding the content of what is being said is difficult for the person, the person then relies heavily on the intonation of the voice and the speaker's body language.

When people are unable to express verbally or feel that their needs are not being acknowledged they may display what is often described as 'attention seeking behaviour'. This type of behaviour is often seen very negatively and as problematic. It is important that health care professionals always pay attention to what the person is trying to tell you by displaying the behaviour. If we consider why the person needs to bang the doors or bite his hand and respond appropriately, it is likely that the behaviour will stop. Of course it is not always as simple as that and being able to identify what the person's behaviour is trying to tell us may need specialist assessment. (*Chapter 4 looks in more detail at behavioural aspects of supporting people with learning disabilities.*)

Reflective Learning Point:

Think about when you have been waiting at a reception desk for attention. What behaviours do you use to attract attention?

Understanding the non-verbal signals is essential especially when caring for people with profound communication difficulties. Family members and carers may be able to give you vital clues to understanding what can sometimes be very subtle, and on occasions, not so subtle clues to what the person is trying to communicate. Some people will have this type of information in a 'Communication Passport' or they may have a pain assessment tool that identifies non-verbal cues to identifying pain when patients are unable to tell you themselves.

Communication passports were first developed by Sally Miller, a speech and language therapist at the University of Edinburgh, and included all aspects of a person's life. They are designed to help a person with limited communication skills to inform those providing services of their needs.

The Disability Distress Assessment Tool (DisDAT 2004) is a tool specifically designed to determine levels of contentment and distress in people with learning disabilities who are unable to express these feelings verbally.

The DisDAT assesses facial signs, appearance, mannerisms and other body language that can be observed and that are known by those who care for the individual to be indicators of contentment and those that indicate distress. These indicators are presented side by side to provide a comparison for the person making an assessment of the patient rather than simply indicating when the person is in distress. By providing a contentment baseline any behaviours that differ from the usual can be compared.

The reliability and validity of the DisDAT is not yet known but, as concluded by Cooper (2009), 'the DisDAT provides a comprehensive assessment when caring for an individual with limited communication', and 'invaluable when used along side a pain protocol for pain relief'. (*Chapter 4 discusses the use of the DisDAT in more detail.*)

Communication Case Study 3 – Non-Verbal Signals – George

George has profound learning disabilities and cerebral palsy. He is in hospital and has been in bed since having surgery on his leg two days ago. It has been noticed that George continually pulls his legs up to his chest and kicks the sheet and blanket off his bed. Because it is quite a warm day he is brought a fan to be placed at the side of his bed and the blanket is removed.

George continues to kick the sheet off his bed so the sheet is removed. However, George does not settle and although he does not appear distressed he continues to lift his knees to his chest.

On reviewing his medical notes it is identified that George has not had his bowels open since admission two days ago. His family says that he always uses the toilet to open his bowels and that he does so daily. George is taken to the toilet and opens his bowels. On return to bed he is settled and the behaviour stops.

This case study shows the importance of comprehensive pre-admission planning around normal daily activities, and having an understanding of what is normal behaviour for an individual. This is the type of information that would be recorded in a prior to admission assessment and a tool such as the DisDAT. (*See Chapter 2 for more detail on pre-admission assessment.*)

For people with very limited communication skills it is most likely that the expression of pain or discomfort will be displayed in a change in behaviour as described in the case study. This example of a behavioural indicator of discomfort was reasonably simple to identify through a process of elimination and information by the carer. However, there may be times when it is not quite as easy to assess what behaviour is communicating. (*Understanding behavioural indicators of distress will be explored in more detail in Chapter 4.*)

For individuals who are able to express themselves verbally it still helps to support what is being said by writing things down or using drawings or diagrams as a prompt; repeating key points; asking the person to explain; or using alternative methods such as tapes.

There are of course other methods of communication that people prefer depending on their needs. Audiotapes and compact discs or video can be an accessible way of providing information to a person who does not have any literacy skills and needs information that they can review time and again. The good thing about using this type of media is that the information can be stopped at any time and go over issues that have not been understood. When using tape to convey a message it is important that the message is short and to the point. It is also important to tell the listener when the message is finished. This is a particularly good method for informing patients about their appointments if they are unable to read an appointment card or letter. (*See later section in this chapter on Tools to aid communication for further information.*)

For more guidance on developing accessible communication you can contact Mencap at: accessibility@mencap.org.uk.

DEVELOPING RELATIONSHIPS WITH PEOPLE WITH A LEARNING DISABILITY

A central factor for health care professionals in working successfully with people with a learning disability is the ability to develop a relationship with the person and really get to know them.

It is only through developing this relationship that you will also develop an understanding of what their learning disability means for them and how it affects their life.

Evidence suggests that patients base their perception of the quality of the care they receive on the approach of the health care professional. Being treated with respect and being spoken to with kindness are high on the priority of how well patients experience their health care.

Reflective Learning Point:

How often have you forgiven the shop assistant for your wait in the queue if they are courteous and helpful when you get to the checkout?

Silverman et al. (2005) outline the following objectives that (Doctors) seek to accomplish in building a relationship with patients:

• Developing rapport to enable the patient to feel understood, valued and supported
• Establishing trust between doctor and patient, laying down the foundation for a therapeutic relationship
• Encouraging an environment that maximises accurate and efficient initiation, information gathering, and explanation and planning
• Enabling supportive counselling as an end in itself
• Developing and maintaining a continuing relationship over time
• Involving the patient so that he or she understands and is comfortable with participating fully in the process of the consultation
• Reducing potential conflict between doctor and patient
• Increasing both the physician's and the patient's satisfaction with the consultation

Whilst this example was written for doctors, the objectives are transferable for any health care professional working in a general hospital. It is possible to achieve all these objectives when working with a person with a learning disability though more creative communication skills may be needed.

Silverman et al. (2005) continue to list the following skills for building the relationship, as illustrated in Box 3.2.

In considering the relationship between a nurse and a patient Tschudin (1991, p. 22) asked nurses to be aware of how their contact with a patient normally starts:

1. The patient is sick; the nurse is healthy.
2. The patient is needy; the nurse can fulfil the need.
3. The patient has only the nurse to relate to; the nurse has other patients and colleagues if she needs a break.
4. The patient is dependent; the nurse has power.
5. The patient is lying down; the nurse is standing over him/her.
6. The patient may have needs of intimate bodily care; the nurse, a stranger, gives this without question.

Tschudin continues to explain that in this kind of helping relationship there is no distinction between physical and psychological care, and that one generally leads to the other, and they

Box 3.2   Skills for building the relationship

Using appropriate non-verbal communication

- *Demonstrates appropriate non-verbal behaviour*: eye contact, facial expression, posture, position, movement, vocal cues, for example rate, volume, intonation
- *Use of notes*: if reads/writes notes or uses computer, does so in a manner that does not interfere with dialogue or rapport
- *Picks up patient's non-verbal cues*: body language, speech, facial expression, checks them out and acknowledges them as appropriate

Developing rapport

- *Acceptance*: accepts legitimacy of patient's views and feelings and is not judgemental
- *Empathy*: uses empathy to communicate understanding and appreciation of the patient's feelings or predicament
- *Support*: expresses concern, understanding, willingness to help, acknowledges coping efforts and appropriate self-care, offers partnership
- *Sensitivity*: deals sensitively with embarrassing and disturbing topics and physical pain, including when associated with physical examination

Involving the patient

- *Sharing of thoughts*: shares thinking with patient to encourage patient involvement
- *Provides rationale*: explains rationale for questions or parts of physical examination
- *Examination:* during physical examination explains process, asks permission

Silverman et al. (2005, p. 122). Reproduced with kind permission of Radcliffe Publishing Ltd.

overlap and interact. She states that 'the challenge to the nurse is to deal with the person not just her problem'. Whilst this is written for nurses it can be equally applied to any other health care professional.

A new approach to developing improved patient experience through patient feedback was the vision of consultant nurse Brigid Reid and her colleagues at East Lancashire Hospitals NHS Trust. Reid identified the need for all health care professionals to understand the implications of behaviour and attitudes in clinical situations and asks, 'What are effective behaviours of staff that enhance the patient experience?' The training scheme devised by Reid and her colleagues helps health care professionals to identify aspects of care that the patient values most. Reid (in Sandiford 2004) says that 'nurses should be like detectives. People give clues the whole time. Picking up on these clues is the key to providing the care the patient is asking for'.

The concept of 'being with the patient' and demonstrating this to the patient by not just physically being present but using active listening skills and providing an environment conducive to safe respectful communication can significantly influence how the patient feels about the interaction. This can be easily demonstrated by adapting our proximity to the patient, for example sitting next to the patient rather than standing by the chair or bed.

More information about 'being with patients' can be found at: www.beingwithpatients@nhs.uk.

Neurberger (1996), cited in Turnbull (1999), suggests that 'Much of what is needed is care and not cure, comfort and not intervention', and that time and space are needed for nurses and patients to form relationships.

Some of the key elements that enhance relationships with patients are:

- Mirroring the behaviour of the patient, smiling.
- Change in posture, gesture, voice tone and breathing. Maintaining a calm non-challenging body posture, avoid crossing arms and rapid bold movements.
- Showing empathy and reflecting feelings.
- Attending and listening.
- Displaying a respectful accepting attitude. This entails not showing any defensiveness towards the person's behaviours or expressions.

Health care professionals need to develop intuitive responses to patient need, focusing on the senses to understand how the patient needs to be responded to. Consider the distressed patient; for some a gentle touch on the arm can be very reassuring, for others a full hug may be what they would want. However, there are individuals who do not want any physical contact and prefer to comfort themselves. Observing the patient can help to identify what level of intervention to take. The person will often offer themselves to you if physical contact is what they need from you.

Reflective Learning Point:

How do you feel about giving physical contact to a patient?
When do you feel it is OK to have contact of this type with a patient?
What are the ethical issues about 'touch' for health care professionals?

The rapport between the health care professional and the patient can be enhanced by developing a mutually acceptable relationship which requires a process of setting boundaries. Some people with learning disabilities may attempt to overstep what may be considered appropriate boundaries by attempting to hug or kiss. Appropriate use of touch must be considered with care. Nelson-Jones (1993) suggests that demonstration of concern in a helping relationship may include touching a patient's hand, arm, shoulder and upper back. It is important that the duration and intensity of the touch is such that it is sufficient to establish concern. Great care must be taken not to allow the touch to hint of any sexual interest. In situations where a patient is inappropriate in their social behaviour it should be gently brought to their attention by altering the greeting with a more appropriate gesture such as touching hands.

The following case study illustrates how a nursing team developed a relationship with someone with severe learning disabilities over a number of years. Figures in brackets in the following case study are references to interviews completed for a research project by Hannon (2003).

Communication Case Study 4 – Developing Relationships – Alan

Alan is a 35-year-old man with a severe learning disability. He uses a wheelchair, and his communication skills are limited. He does not have any behaviour problems. Alan needs full support with personal care, and has been in hospital on many occasions previously. Alan had a planned admission every 4 weeks, and was well known and accepted on the ward.

Alan was supported by his carer, a registered nurse (learning disability), and a community LD nurse, who completed the pre-admission assessment with them. His carer stayed with him, and had previous experience of hospital admission with him. The community nurse has 19 years' experience, and has known Alan for 7 years. She has previous experience of supporting people with a learning disability during hospital admission.

The ward sister, who has 25 years' nursing experience, cared for him. The sister did some training as a cadet nurse at a local learning disability hospital, and had known Alan since he was a child.

His carer felt that nurses who had experience within learning disability services showed a better understanding of his needs. She said, [3.151–156] 'They are a bit frightened are general nurses and it's like the unknown really. How to approach them, how to handle them, and they can't understand'.

A person-centred, multi-disciplinary care plan had been developed over a number of years that was fully responsive and meeting his needs. He needed minimal support from carers, even when he had to stay overnight. Hospital staff were confident in supporting him. Alan was happy with care received.

His carer highlighted that, like many other people with a learning disability, he was brought up in a hospital environment and seeing nurses in uniform was [3.180] 'Something very comfortable for him really'. Alan's carer felt that he can sometimes seem [3.210] 'A bit lost and he is happy for that emotional support' that the carer provided. She also felt that he needed [3.222] 'Somebody to talk to on his level'.

The community nurse thought it was useful to have a named hospital nurse for liaison, and for Alan to go to if he needed anything. [1.74] 'Not just physical needs, it was about psychological and emotional needs'.

Communication was an issue; carers understand what Alan needs but know that he is not able to ask for them. [3.259] 'It's obvious he's in a wheelchair, there's a lot of obvious things, but it isn't obvious that he isn't able to communicate just as good as they think he might be able to'.

The ward sister felt the main things hospital staff needed to know was [4.18] 'How much do (people with learning disabilities) understand, and how much can they do for themselves', and [4.60] 'How much they can actually communicate and how, in what way will they communicate'.

Everyone agreed this was a successful admission, and no problems were highlighted.

An important factor to consider in developing relationships with people with a learning disability is the need for the person to be considered an equal partner in the health care process. The evidence base highlights that health care professionals in general hospitals are often unsure about how much a person with a learning disability can do for themselves and how much they need help with. This can often lead to staff under or over-protecting people.

Under-protecting people can lead to situations where health needs are not met, some of which are outlined in the Ombudsman Report 'Six Lives' (Parliamentary and Health Service Ombudsman 2009) and are explored further in the ethical issues section of Chapter 6.

Many health care professionals have the view that people with a learning disability are 'eternal children' and take a paternalistic approach to their interactions with them. In transactional analysis terms, using the 'ego state' model of personality, over-protecting people would be described as a 'parent–child relationship', when the aim for health care professionals should be to develop an 'adult–adult relationship' wherever possible.

Transactional analysis (TA) is a 'contractual and goal orientated psychotherapy' 'rooted within the humanistic tradition' explains Robinson, in Jukes and Aldridge (2006, p. 157). She describes how TA values the whole person, body, mind and spirit, and how TA techniques can be implemented with people with a learning disability helping them to make significant changes and developments in their lives, and providing benefit to people presenting with emotional distress.

In TA, communication skills are identified as 'transactions' and the interpretation and understanding of these contributes to providing an explanation for psychological stability and disturbance. Whilst this is a highly skilled intervention, particularly when used with people with a learning disability, health care professionals can be aware of the importance of communicating with people as an equal (adult to adult), helping them to listen, understand and plan appropriate interventions.

Robinson recommends the following books for people who may be interested in developing a wider knowledge of TA:

- Stewart I and Joines V (1987) *TA Today*. Lifespace Publishing, Kegworth.
- Stewart I (1996) *Transactional Analysis Counselling in Action*, 2nd edition. Sage, London.
- Joines V and Stewart I (2002) *Personality Adaptations*. Lifespace Publishing, Kegworth.

COMMUNICATING WITH PEOPLE WITH A LEARNING DISABILITY

Effective communication is the key to working with people with a learning disability. The ability to connect with the person and relate to them on their own level requires skilled and sensitive interaction from health care professionals in order to understand what the person needs, and the ability to think creatively about how you can get your message across.

Reflective Learning Point:

Think how you would explain a complex medical procedure to someone with limited communication skills – how would you tell them what you are going to do?

Cumella and Martin (2000) report that 'Both nationally and internationally research has shown that communication difficulties between healthcare providers and patients with learning disabilities pose huge barriers for this group accessing effective and appropriate healthcare'.

Health care and treatment requires the cooperation of the patient in both their consent to treatment taking place, and in the delivery of the treatment itself. For people with learning disabilities who do not understand what is happening to them, due to breakdown in communication, this can have catastrophic effects. The fear and stress experienced as a result of not being fully prepared for any procedure can lead to non-cooperation. Sowney and Barr (2007) identify the consequences of staff inadvertently causing harm through their inactions rather than actions.

Effective communication is essential to providing quality health care. Sowney and Barr (2007) highlighted that 'Communicating with people with a learning disability was perceived to be the biggest challenge within accident and emergency environments'. The challenges in communication were associated with difficulties assessing health care needs, informing patients of their health status, and in seeking consent. They identified that health care professionals in emergency departments had three main difficulties in communicating with patients with learning disabilities. The first being a lack of knowledge of the nature of learning disability; second, having time to assess and respond appropriately to communication needs due to a need to move the patient speedily through the process; and third, understanding non-verbal communication especially in relation to communicating pain. (*Chapter 4 discusses in detail how behavioural assessment can assist in the identification of pain in patients who have learning disabilities.*)

Health care professionals concern about obtaining consent prior to procedures and their reluctance to proceed without someone to take responsibility for the decision making, for example next of kin has caused inappropriate delays in treatment for some individuals in the past. It is vitally important, therefore, that health care professionals have a clear understanding of not only how to implement the Mental Capacity Act (Department of Health 2005) (see Chapter 5) but also how to communicate effectively with their patient.

An individual's communication needs should not be considered in isolation. Money, in Abudarham and Hurd (2002, p. 86), highlights that it is important to consider the communication in the context of 'how staff and service users communicate (means), why they communicate (reasons) and with whom, where, and when do they communicate (opportunities)'. She suggests a number of approaches to managing communication needs based on either a direct approach; developing the individual's communication abilities, an indirect approach; developing opportunities for communication through training for carers or environmental programmes, or a combination of both of these.

Communication skills

To understand the communication issues faced by people with learning disabilities it is important to understand the skills required to communicate effectively. In their book *Teaching and Learning Communication Skills in Medicine* Kurtz et al. (1998) demonstrated that:

- The doctor–patient relationship is central to clinical practice.
- Communication is a core clinical skill, an essential component of clinical competence.
- Communication skills need to be taught and learned.
- Specific teaching and learning methods are required in communication skills training.

In the companion book Silverman et al. (2005, p. 8) outlined that 'the prize on offer from communication skills training is improved clinical performance' and highlighted the following key concepts:

- Communication is not just 'being nice' but produces a more effective consultation for both patient and doctor.

- Effective consultation significantly improves:
  - Accuracy, efficiency and supportiveness
  - Health outcomes for the patients
  - Satisfaction for both patient and doctor
  - The therapeutic relationship
- Communication bridges the gap between evidence-based medicine and working with individual patients.

Silverman et al. (2005, p. 58) outline the following key objectives when gathering information in medical interviews:

- Explore the patient's problems to discover the biomedical perspective, the patient's perspective and the background information
- Ensure that information gathered is accurate, complete and mutually understood (establishing common ground)
- Ensure that patients feel listened to, and that their information and views are welcomed and valued (confirmation)
- Continue to develop a supportive environment and a collaborative relationship
- Structure the consultation to ensure efficient information gathering and to enable the patient to understand and be overtly involved in where the interview is going and why

When you first meet someone with a learning disability it is important to talk directly to them in a respectful manner. Do not automatically assume they have communication/comprehension problems until you get to know them better. If it becomes apparent that the person has limited communication then involve the carer – in this way no one is embarrassed or offended. It is important to talk to the person as an adult not as a child – though you may need to adapt some of the words used to accommodate their level of understanding.

Hannon (2003) found that whilst most people with a learning disability felt that hospital staff spoke directly to them, some felt that they spoke to the person supporting them instead. One person reported that 'the Doctor just walks past me, he didn't speak to me'.

The skills and opportunities outlined by Cogher (2005) that we need for effective communication are illustrated in the language skills model in Figure 3.3.

In considering the key components of the model above, the main barriers to the communication cycle for people with a learning disability in health care situations are:

- Cognitive deficits; not understanding what is being said or not having the ability to process the information
- The opportunity to learn and use language skills
- Hearing impairment
- Attention deficits; difficulty with concentration
- Inability to move the mouth in a coordinated way to make speech sounds
- Pragmatic competence in social situations

Some clients may have difficulties with expressing and understanding social language. This often relates to how a person interacts rather than what they are saying, and may include areas such as body language, facial expression and proximity. People with a learning disability may not have developed an awareness of the social skills required in different situations due to limited life experiences.

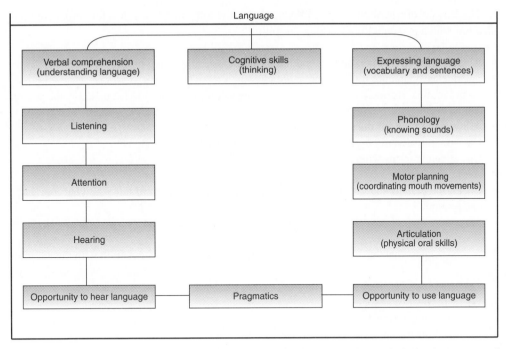

Fig. 3.3   The language skills model. From Grant et al. © 2005, Reproduced with the kind permission of Open University Press. All rights reserved.

Health care professionals need a key range of skills in order to communicate effectively with people with a learning disability such as:

- Active listening
- No use of jargon
- Ask questions to clarify understanding and check preferences
- Ability to provide simple explanations of complex treatment interventions
- Verbal and non-verbal communication skills and knowledge
- Eye contact
- Active interaction
- Positive regard for the individual
- Open and friendly approach
- Sensitive to individual needs
- Confidence in approaching and dealing with the person
- Understanding of how the learning disability impacts on the individual
- Use of person-centred approaches

Hannon (2003) quoted a person with a learning disability who was admitted to hospital who said 'Communication is important; people may feel angry or upset if they didn't understand what was happening, or couldn't speak up. It can be helpful to get a family member to communicate for them. Some people may not speak English very well, or don't understand the words the doctors' use'.

The Royal College of Nursing (2006) highlights the following key points for verbal communication with a person with a learning disability:

- Always speak to the person first and not to the person supporting them
- Speak clearly and not too fast and avoid jargon
- To reduce anxiety and build confidence, start by asking some questions you know the person can answer
- Allow more time for the person to think
- Use straightforward language and short, plain sentences
- Use concrete terms wherever possible – and avoid abstracts
- Avoid abbreviations
- Check the person understands what you have said and ask them to tell you what they have understood
- Make sure the conversation has a clear beginning, middle and end

They also suggest that the same guidance is applied to written communication with the addition of:

- Write as you would speak
- Use consistent words throughout
- Use symbols for numbers (9) not words (nine)
- Use one photograph to support each idea
- Refer to the person as 'you' and the service as 'we'
- Use a minimum font size of 14

Active listening

When interacting with patients, health care professionals may not always be listening attentively to what they are saying. We may be distracted, thinking about other things, or thinking about what you are going to say next. Active listening is a structured way of listening and responding to others. It focuses attention on the speaker. Suspending one's own frame of reference and suspending judgment are important in order to fully attend to the speaker.

It is important to observe the other person's behaviour and body language. Having the ability to interpret a person's body language allows the listener to develop a more accurate understanding of the speaker's words. This could be described as the listener is 'listening for feelings'. Thus, rather than merely repeating what the speaker has said, the active listener might describe the underlying emotion, for example 'you seem to feel angry' or 'you seem to feel frustrated'.

The following information about active listening can be obtained from the Samaritans website at: http://www.samaritans.org/default.aspx?page=7508.

Active Listening

We can all think of situations where we found it hard to talk about something that was troubling us. Difficult, painful or just embarrassing situations which we found almost impossible to speak to someone about. Imagine you have got a colleague or friend who needs to get something difficult off their chest. How do you get them to open up?

Active listening is a way of listening which helps people talk through their problems, however difficult to put into words they find it. With active listening, although you actually do some talking, you are really acting as a sounding board. Whatever you say does not influence what the other person has to say – it just helps them to talk. Here are some suggestions to help you actively listen in a conversation:

1. *Open questions*: Rather than asking questions which only require a yes or no answer, try and ask open questions. For example, instead of saying: 'Has this been going on a long time?' ask 'How long has this been going on?' That way, instead of closing the conversation down into a yes or no response, you open it out and encourage the other person to keep talking. Another good example to remember is instead of saying 'is everything ok?' you can ask 'how are things going?'
2. *Summarising*: This helps to show that you have listened to, and understood, what is being said. For example, 'So you're feeling very stressed by your work, but you still love your job'. (The listener may also 'paraphrase' the speaker's words – simply stating what was said in a slightly different way.)
3. *Reflecting*: Repeating back a word or phrase can encourage people to go on. If someone says, 'So it's been really difficult recently,' you can keep the conversation going simply by repeating 'Difficult. . .'
4. *Clarifying*: We all skirt around or gloss over the most difficult things. If we can avoid saying them, we will. If the person you are speaking with glosses over an important point, saying 'Tell me more about. . .', or '. . . sounds a difficult area for you' can help them clarify the points, not only for you, but for themselves. It sounds obvious, but a 'Yes', 'Go on', or 'I see' can really give some much-needed encouragement.
5. *Reacting*: You do not have to be completely neutral. If whoever you are talking with has been having an absolutely dreadful time of it, some sympathy and understanding is vital. 'That must have been difficult', 'You've had an awful time' – this really helps.

All of this sounds quite simple. And it is. All you are doing is listening, and from time to time giving responses which encourage the other person to keep on talking. **That is often the key – get them to keep on talking**.

Active listening is used in a wide variety of situations, including health care professionals talking to patients. Although there are some barriers that may affect the flow of communication between individuals, the benefits of active listening include getting people to open up, avoiding misunderstandings, resolving conflict and building trust. In a medical context, benefits may include increased patient satisfaction, improving cross-cultural communication, improved outcomes or decreased litigation.

How to identify if your patient has communication difficulties?

In some cases it may be perfectly apparent that the person you are talking to is unable to understand what you are saying to them. Sometimes the person supporting the patient may want to do all the talking and not give you the opportunity to assess how much they can understand and express for themselves. It is extremely important especially when the health care professional is attempting to establish whether or not the patient is able to understand the proposed care or treatment that the patient's communication ability is assessed appropriately.

There are a number of clues that can help identify communication difficulties that can be picked up by making general conversation. By spending a short amount of time developing a relationship with the patient and opening up a channel of communication there will be elements of the interaction that may help to identify communication deficits.

Some indicators of communication difficulties may be:

- *The person always goes for first or second of any two choices*: This is often due to auditory memory difficulties, for example 'Do you want tea, coffee or something else?' The person will always take tea, understanding the first thing you said, or may just repeat the last thing you tell them.
- *The person says associative things*: If you ask about an issue that the person has experience of they may relate what you are asking to this experience. Care is needed to ensure that this link is relevant.
- *Acquiescence*: Giving the answers that the person thinks you want to hear or just going along with what they are told.
- *Keeps talking, or keeps talking about own topics*: Talking about issues that you have understanding of develops your social networks and relationships. Patients who talk about unrelated issues probably highlight an inability to know how to talk to you in their current situation. This could also suggest that the person is feeling vulnerable and finds talking about thing he understands comforting and distracting from the presenting issue.
- *The person has word-finding difficulties*: For example, uses 'You know', 'um',' thingy', 'the wotsit' etc.
- *Using words without really understanding them*: Depending on the life experiences of the patient, this will influence the conversational skills and vocabulary that the person uses. The use of complex vocabulary can often cause confusion for health care professionals and a belief that the person has a greater level of comprehension than they actually have.
- *The person has auditory memory difficulties*: For example, repeats what you say back.
- *Person is distracted or confused if two people talking at the same time.*
- *Says yes to everything*! People with learning disabilities can often feel the need to please. Equally there are individuals that will say 'no' to everything. This can also because they are unable to think through the options given to them or be able to identify what those options may be.
- *Person asks the same questions over and over*: This behaviour usually suggests that the person has not understood the answer that was given previously. It is important to be consistent in the words used when providing feedback to questions. Not only consistent in the answer given but in the words that are used when answering.
- *Says things like 'Ask my staff'*: This can be a common response. People with learning disabilities are often very used to staff speaking for them. This may be because the person does not understand what you are asking, but equally it may be because they do not have the skills to articulate their answers, not that they do not have an answer to give.
- *Can talk about everyday things but not emotions or opinions*: Emotions and opinions can be difficult to articulate and are much more difficult to identify.
- *Takes things literally, does not understand humour*: This is particularly common with people with autistic spectrum disorder.
- *Person looks blank or gets anxious when asked to make a choice*: Remember to give the person time to give a response; it may take them sometime to process the information. Do not try to rush a response or be tempted to give the information in an alternative way as this could cause more confusion or anxiety.

- *Person answers previous question or is still talking about previous topic*: Be aware that for some people it may take longer than usual to process the question that you have given them. Look for thinking clues, 'um's' and looking to the floor or to the ceiling can suggest that the person is processing your question. Some people can take more than a minute to answer a question.
- *The carer tells you that the person 'understands everything you say'*: It is always important to check this out. As discussed previously, carers can often underestimate or overestimate what the person understands. However, if the situation is new to the person it is likely that they may have more difficulty understanding new information and may need more time to process the information.

A simple tool to test comprehension is to ask the person to tell you what they have understood of what you have told them. This will allow you to assess for evidence of misunderstanding of certain words or statements. Indicators that the person has an understanding of the verbal information put to them can be identified by the person are as follows:

- Showing signs of listening, not being distracted, holding eye contact. Some people, however, may not display these behaviours, individuals with autism for example
- Use of reinforcing behaviours like nodding or responding with 'I see', 'ah ha'
- Responding with appropriate questions or reflecting back
- Seeking clarification
- Appropriately maintaining the conversation. Not interrupting and responding to cues for responses

When an individual is unable to communicate verbally, it is necessary to observe the non-verbal signals that suggest understanding such as nodding, pointing, smiling, gestures that are known to indicate yes or no. Similar indicators in the assessment of accessible information can be utilised by checking out what the person can tell you about the pictures or symbols mean to them. The individual's family or carers may be helpful in establishing these indicators.

The National Patient Safety Agency (NPSA 2004) highlighted that people with learning disabilities state that they feel that they are not given enough time to speak up for themselves. People with learning disabilities may require longer than the usual consultation time allocated to a patient to allow for the additional time to ensure the patient is fully informed and has the opportunity to express themselves. The person may not be listening because they are in pain, tired, or experiencing mental health issues. It is also important to look out for signs of hearing loss, especially in people with Down's syndrome

The British Medical Association (BMA 2007) stresses that poor listening and communication skills by health care professionals can increase the likelihood of diagnostic overshadowing. The BMA also suggests that it is often poor organisation and lack of resources that lead to poor communication between the health care professional and the patient. Communication can be improved by identifying the barriers and utilising resources to overcome those barriers.

Speech and language therapists are the key health care professionals in assessing and working with communication needs for people with a learning disability. Through their careful assessment they will be able to identify the exact nature and severity of the communication needs of the individual. The assessment will include identifying any potential causes of the communication needs, which is important to consider when developing communication approaches. The assessment will identify the individual's strengths and areas for development, which will also highlight possible approaches that are more likely to be successfully used. Repeated assessment and monitoring over time will enable any progress to be noted and evaluate the effectiveness of any interventions used.

Suggestibility and acquiescence

There is evidence to suggest that people with learning disabilities, in particular those with mild learning disability, are particularly susceptible to suggestion in interview situations. The work of Clare and Gudjonsson (reported in Kelly 2000) in relation to people with learning disabilities within the criminal justice system reflects some of the issues for people with a learning disability in health care consultations.

Acquiescence is the tendency to say 'yes' to 'yes/no' questioning. Clare and Gudjonsson found that acquiescent responding is related to poor intellectual skills. They also noted that people with mild learning disabilities were much more susceptible to leading questions and were more likely to confabulate (i.e. invent past experiences).

In the authors' experience there have been concerning moments in consulting rooms when supporting patients who have agreed to suggested symptoms described by the doctor that do not bear any relation to the experience of the patient. Although it is vitally important to listen to the patient's experience when assessing the symptoms of a presenting condition, it is also important to balance this out with taking an accurate medical history, and completing any necessary analysis and checks to confirm symptoms.

Although closed questions (e.g. where is the pain?) are useful for clarifying specific points, open questioning (e.g. can you tell me about the pain you have been having?) encourages the person to tell you more about how the symptoms have been affecting their life, and can help you explore and pick up more clues about what is happening.

Therefore, it is vitally important when questioning patients who have learning disabilities that the consultation does not heavily rely on the use of closed or leading questions that can result in unreliable assessment. If you think the person is acquiescing ask the same question later but in a different way.

We can sometimes be misled by what appears to be expressive language and comprehension when for example the person is able to give what appears to be a knowledgeable response to a question when assessing understanding in consent to treatment situations. Some people, in particular people with autism, are able to remember detailed information sometimes even long conversations, and are able to repeat the conversation back word for word. This is known as echolalia. Echolalia is the repetition of words spoken without the understanding of what the words mean. Some individuals will be able to remember the conversation or statement for some time and be able to repeat it over and over again.

Responding to communication needs

It is important that health care professionals develop the skills to respond to the communication needs of people with learning disabilities. Having recognised that the person has communication difficulties it may be necessary to solicit advice from family, carers or other professionals to ensure that an appropriate method of communicating with the person is established. Being aware of and adjusting your verbal communication skills can make a real difference when communicating with people with learning disabilities.

Some tips for improving communication are:

- Check if the person has any sensory impairments that may affect their ability to hear or communicate.
- Pay attention to slowing the pace at which you talk. For some people it takes longer for them to process the information you are giving them. By talking quickly they can miss out on the important part of the sentence.
- Allow time for the person to process information. Do not assume they are not able to reply if they do not answer straightaway.
- Use everyday words rather than technical terms. It is extremely important to establish the vocabulary that is understandable to the person. Use words such as 'hurt' and 'sore' instead of 'tender' and 'discomfort'.
- Check the terminology the person uses – for example tummy or stomach. Point to the relevant part of the body to show what you are talking about.
- Avoid euphemisms – for example do not say 'does it hurt when you spend a penny?' It is much better to say 'does it hurt when you have a wee?' Commonly patients are asked if they have had their 'bowels open'. Although it may feel unprofessional or embarrassing to use a word that is more familiar to the person, it ensures that the person understands what you are referring to.
- Use gestures and facial expressions to support what you are saying.
- Always face the person you are talking to.
- Think about the length and complexity of the sentence. The use of negatives in sentences can easily be misunderstood. Avoid whenever possible the use of words like 'don't' and statements such as 'it isn't time for' or 'there isn't any'. Keep sentences to a minimum to maximise the person's ability to understand what is being said to them.
- Always check that understanding has occurred.

Reflective Learning Point:

Consider the request: 'Go to the changing room and put on the gown and your slippers and then come back to the waiting area'.

It would be easier for the person to be able to follow this direction without error if the sentence was divided. This may require the person being taken to the changing area and told to 'put on the gown' and then when they have done that to be told 'Now come back to the waiting room'.

How many times has the patient stayed in the changing room because they have forgotten where you told them to go!

In most cases an appropriate method of communication can be identified. If the person uses an alternative form of communication it is important that everyone knows how to use this. Even for individuals who are able to express themselves verbally it often still helps to support what is being said by writing things down or using drawings or diagrams as a prompt, repeating key points, and asking the person to explain what is happening so you can check their understanding. However, if the situation is complex and the person needs more specialist support, the learning disability service often have speech and language therapists who are skilled in the assessment of communication difficulties and the development of accessible information. (*See also section later in this chapter on Tools to aid communication.*)

Overcoming barriers to communication

It is very important to ensure that the person has every opportunity to hear what you are saying to them. Always ensure that the environment is as quiet and distraction free as possible and that if the person has a hearing impairment that any hearing aid and the loop system, if installed in your department, is switched on.

The DDA (Department of Health 1995) makes it unlawful for service providers to discriminate against disabled people. The DDA applies to nearly all service providers of which health care providers such as hospitals and clinics are included. Since 1999, services have been required to make reasonable adjustments to the services they provide to ensure that people with disabilities have equal access to care and treatment. These adjustments include meeting the needs of people with hearing, sight and communication difficulties by:

- Installing induction loop systems for people with hearing impairment
- Providing interpreters for people who use sign language
- Providing information in accessible formats – large print, easy read, pictorial, Braille and audio versions of all information resources

The DDA also recommends training for all staff to enable them to support people with disabilities appropriately.

Sir Jonathon Michaels (2008), in his executive summary, stated that 'There is insufficient attention given to making reasonable adjustments to support the delivery of equal treatment, as required by the Disability Discrimination Act. Adjustments are not always made to allow for communication problems, difficulty in understanding (cognitive impairment), or the anxieties and preferences of individuals regarding their treatment'. He goes on in his recommendations to say that 'The Department of Health should immediately amend Core Standards for Better Health, to include an explicit reference to the requirement to make "reasonable adjustments" to the provision and delivery of service to vulnerable groups, in accordance with the disability equality legislation'.

Reflective Learning Point:

It should therefore be in the minds of all health care professionals when considering the needs of patients in relation to communication that they pay due attention to the requirements of the Disability Discrimination Act.

A copy can be obtained from: http://www.dwp.gov.uk/employers/dda.

The NPSA in 2004 raised concerns that there is a lack of accessible information informing patients about their medication. They not only stated that accessible information is important in the management of safe medicine administration, but also highlighted the need for all information for patients to be provided in an accessible format. (*Examples of accessible information can be found later in this chapter and also in Chapter 2.*)

TOOLS TO AID COMMUNICATION

Although some people with a learning disability may have communication tools that they use in their daily life, this may not always meet their needs during their stay in hospital. This is often the case because staff in the hospital are not familiar with the model of communication used. How the person communicates, their level of understanding, and how you should explain things to them should all be identified and agreed prior to the hospital admission wherever possible. When it is identified that the person you are communicating with has communication difficulties it may be necessary to consider an augmentative or alternative form of communication.

Augmentative and alternative forms of communication

Augmentative and alternative communication (AAC) systems are usually implemented to provide support to enhance communication where a person with physical or cognitive disabilities is unable to rely on verbal speech as their main means of communication. They provide individuals with a functional means of communication and anything that increases the effectiveness of spoken communication, or can be used as a non-verbal means of communication included in this description.

The majority of people who use AAC employ a mixture of aided and unaided communication systems. Unaided communication uses the person's own body and is usually in the form of gestures and/or signing. Aided systems use equipment in addition to the person's own body. This equipment can often be quite simple though advances in information technology have led to the development of numerous high-tech computer-based communication systems.

Light (1989) described communicative competence for individuals using AAC as 'The quality of being functionally adequate in daily communication, or of having sufficient knowledge, judgement, and skill to communicate'. She outlined the four communication competencies for individuals as:

- *Linguistic competence*: an adequate level of mastery of the linguistic code
- *Operational competence*: the user must also develop the technical skills to operate the system
- *Social competence*: the user of an AAC system must also possess knowledge, judgement and skill in the social rules of communication
- *Strategic competence*: to make the best of what they do know and can do

Total communication philosophy (TCP) is an approach that includes the complementary use of speech, signs and symbols to enable people with learning disabilities to understand and express themselves to their maximum potential. Every form of communication of which a person is capable of using is used. TCP uses a variety of augmentative and alternative modes of communication such as gestures, signs and symbols which will be explored in more detail within this section.

For some clients whom we work with, communicating through the spoken language may not be an option. We may need to use some other formal means of communication (e.g. communication aids, signing [Makaton], objects of reference). We need to consider each person as an individual, their sensory preferences, additional needs, what is functional and meaningful to them in their lives.

Use of signing and gesturing

Facial expression, body language and gestures are universal ways of expressing ourselves. As discussed previously, how we present ourselves non-verbally has a greater impact on how the person understands us, and our message is not just based on the words we use. How often do you use these non-verbal skills to get your message across?

Reflective Learning Point:

Think about the last time you were on holiday and you could not speak the local language, or you were in a noisy crowded place when you are trying to get your message across. How did this make you feel? What would have helped you to communicate?

Signing is a slightly more formal use of gesture. Signing is often used to help people with a learning disability enhance their spoken language and provide another method of communicating. One of the most common signing systems used for people with learning disabilities is *Makaton* signing.

Makaton is a multi-modal language programme devised by a speech and language therapist, Margaret Walker, in 1972/3. Makaton is used extensively all over the UK for supporting children and adults with a learning disability to develop their communication, language and literacy skills. It has a vocabulary of signs for use with children and adults with a wide range of communication needs and their interactive partners. Makaton has also been adapted for use in 40 other countries.

The essential features of Makaton are that it has a core vocabulary of 450 concepts and a resource vocabulary of over 7,000 concepts. It is used with speech, signs and/or symbols and concentrates on key words and can be used at a variety of levels from single words to full sentences and conversation. The majority of signs used in the UK with Makaton are taken from British Sign Language (BSL), the cultural language of the UK deaf community. The symbols are unique to Makaton.

The Makaton language programme is widely used by people with learning disabilities, yet Hannon (2003) found in her research study that no one at the hospital had heard of it. One of the people with a learning disability involved in the study, when talking about how health care professionals could communicate with him about health interventions explained, 'Some people don't understand, completely don't understand, so if they had Makaton it would be easier for them to understand. Or the symbols can do it, anything like a picture or something. A picture and they will understand what it is'.

Some signs and symbols are easily recognisable, and if the health care professional is caring for a patient who uses Makaton or BSL, it is supportive to the patient to learn some familiar signs and symbols, or signs and symbols that will be important when needing to communicate treatment information to them. The patient and their family or carer will probably be able to give information about the signs to use. You could also contact your speech and language department or learning disability liaison nurse.

Figure 3.4 shows some of the commonly used Makaton signs.

More Signs and symbols and information about Makaton can be found at: www.makaton.org.

Aided communication

As outlined earlier, aided communication involves the use of equipment in addition to the person's own body. This includes the use of objects, pictures, photographs, written or graphic symbols, communication boards, charts and books.

Advances in information technology have led to the development of numerous high-tech computer-based communication systems too complex to discuss in detail here. Some people with a learning disability have access to a variety of electronic equipment, including portable computers with special software, communication aids that produce speech or text, adapted keyboards and pointer control systems. If someone is admitted to hospital using any of this type of equipment it is vital for the health care team to become familiar with its use prior to the admission.

More commonly you may see people with a learning disability who use some form of communication book. This may include any combination of signs, symbols, pictures or photographs that they use to express their needs. It could be as simple as a picture of a cup that someone can point to when they want a drink, or a photograph of a body part that they can use to show you where it is hurting. This is a useful option to consider when preparing accessible information to tell someone about a particular procedure for example. (*See also example of accessible treatment plan later in this chapter.*)

Objects of reference

This term refers to using objects as a means of communication, for example a spoon to represent dinner, sponge to represent bath time, etc. The use of an object to aid understanding is particularly helpful when prompting regular routines such as eating and drinking, personal care and activities. Objects of reference can aid memory, encourage or initiate communication, and introduce and expand choice for the individual.

The benefits of using objects of reference to aid communication are that the object is permanent and identical each time. For example, the patients' own cup to inform that they are going to have a drink or for the patient to tell you that they want a drink. The object refers to a particular activity and conveys a message, in this case that a drink is coming or is wanted. Objects are also more accessible for those people who have hearing or visual impairment, those who cannot use any form of sign language or who have difficulty following spoken language. Using objects effectively to provide a method of communicating can be motivating for the individual and positively enhances the quality of the person's life.

The health care professional can use the object of reference to alert the patient to an activity, for example giving the patient a sponge when it is time to be washed. The object of reference can give the patient control over activities by them accepting the object when agreeing to the activity or offering the object to the health care professional when requesting help or intervention. This can be useful to timetable or sequence events. For objects of reference to be effective they must be relevant to the person. It is important that both health care professional and patient understand the meaning of the object of reference and that it is used appropriately.

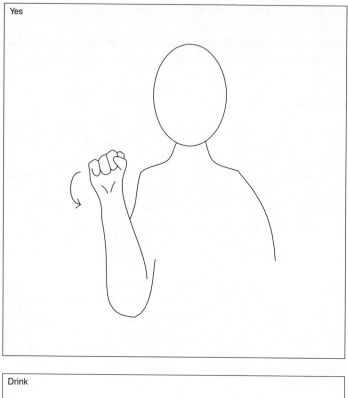

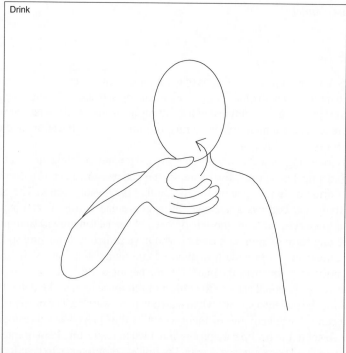

Fig. 3.4   Some useful Makaton signs. Makaton symbols and line drawings of signs are reproduced with permission from the Makaton Charity.

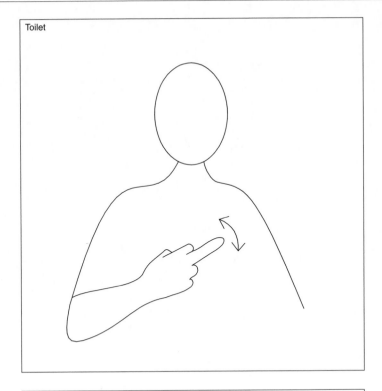

Toilet

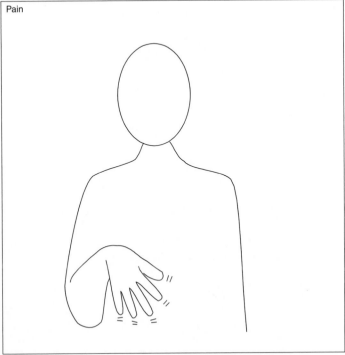

Pain

Fig. 3.4 (Continued)

Nurse

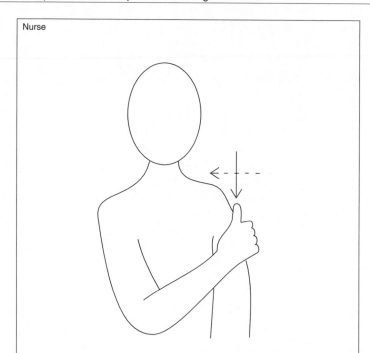

Doctor

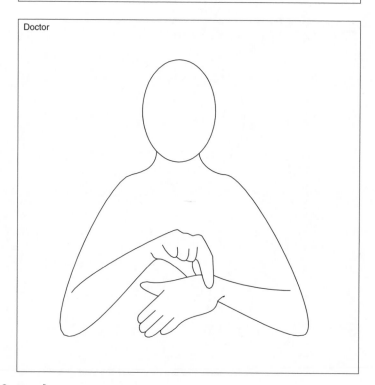

Fig. 3.4   (Continued)

Consistency is the key to the successful use of objects of reference. Frequent and consistent use helps the individual to build links between the activity and the object. This also enables more than one person using any object to help learning and communication to take place.

The following case study illustrates the use of an object of reference on the ward:

Communication Case Study 5 – Object of Reference – Lauren

Lauren has profound learning disabilities and is unable to communicate verbally. The ward staff are having difficulties encouraging Lauren to take fluids and are concerned that she will require intravenous fluids.

Lauren's home care staff use her red beaker cup at home whenever she has a drink, so they bring it to the ward for Lauren to use. Lauren also bangs the cup on her table when she is thirsty to alert staff that she wants to drink.

By simply providing Lauren with a familiar object she is able to communicate her need and understands that the drink provided is for her.

When explaining a procedure or treatment to a patient it can sometimes be helpful to use objects to aid comprehension and understanding, by showing the patient the equipment to be used before hand. Care of course needs to be taken in deciding the appropriateness of the patient viewing equipment as the intention is not to cause more anxiety.

The following case study demonstrates that modelling a procedure as part of the assessment of capacity prior to the procedure being carried out can be helpful in establishing how much the patient understands of what is going to happen.

Communication Case Study 6 – Object of Reference – Peter

Peter has autism and moderate learning disabilities. He is admitted to a hospital due to pain and swelling in his abdomen. Peter is extremely anxious and reluctant to allow anyone to examine him. Peter is told that he is going to have a special test using a camera to look into his bowel. Peter refuses to allow the endoscopy procedure.

The issue for Peter was his understanding of what it would mean to have a camera put into his back passage. Peter's understanding of a camera is the one his father uses when they go on holiday. To help Peter understand the difference between the equipment he understands as a camera, and the endoscopy equipment, required a visit to the endoscopy department to view the equipment. It was decided that using the actual object rather than a photograph was the best aid to communication because, as for many people with autism, he had difficulties relating photographic images to real-life situations. Peter was happy to proceed following this visit.

Objects of reference are really useful when used sensitively in this way, and are particularly helpful for preparing the patient when the procedure is ready to proceed. It is important to consider when choosing to use objects to aid understanding that the object is real and meaningful, and wherever possible you should use a real-life object in the activity. The use of abstract objects, miniature objects or objects with shared features should only be considered as an exception when the real object is not available.

The use of images to improve communication

Photographs, diagrams, pictures and symbols

Mencap (2002), in its guidelines for accessible writing 'Am I making myself clear?', identifies that photographs were the most popular kind of image. However, whether you use photographs, pictures or symbols the importance is that the image best explains the text to the reader.

Photographs, diagrams, pictures and symbols can be really useful for people who have:

- Difficulty understanding spoken language
- Memory difficulties
- Limited or unintelligible speech
- Rigid behaviour patterns
- Limited literacy skills

Photographs, diagrams, pictures and symbols can be used to:

- *Increase understanding*: give more information than spoken word
- *Provide prompts*: inform what's happening, any change of routine
- *Aid memory*: they remain, whereas the spoken word fades
- *Empower*: provide a means of expression and making choices
- Motivate and maintain interest
- Create notices and labels
- Keep a record of items discussed at meetings and for correspondence

Images can be particularly effective when used as a memory aid, especially when the person has items to remember or a sequence of events. For some people their anxiety is raised by having a procedure and also feeling unsure about what is going to happen. Flash cards with images of the sequence of events can help remind the person what is going to happen and reduce the anxiety of feeling unsure of what will happen next.

Communication Case Study 7 – Use of Flash Cards – Andrea

Andrea was always very anxious when she needed any medical intervention. She would cry, become distressed and hyperventilate at the sight of a health care professional. It was felt by her carer that the distress was based on her anxiety of not understanding what would happen. Andrea needed to have a procedure that would require her cooperation over a number of hours and that she would need to keep as calm as possible.

Andrea was provided with a series of flash cards that would inform her of the treatment process to help her understand what would happen in sequence. Andrea was able to talk through the cards with her carer prior to admission to the hospital. Although Andrea was unable to consent to the procedure because she was unable to retain the information long enough to make a decision about her treatment, the flash cards would help her have an understanding of what would happen while she was admitted.

During the treatment Andrea and her carer followed the sequence of flash cards at each step of her treatment. The flash cards helped to minimise Andrea's anticipatory anxiety during the admission and she was able to have her treatment without becoming tearful or distressed.

Photographs can be helpful when a person has difficulty making choices, though it is important that the options are kept to a minimum. Decision making can be difficult if too many choices are offered at the same time. Limiting the choices to be made at any one time can be helpful especially if the person has memory problems and/or difficulties understanding complex information.

The following case study demonstrates how notices and labels that are accompanied by a picture or symbol can empower the person to be more independent in their environment.

Communication Case Study 8 – Use of symbols – John

John is a patient on a medical ward. John is a quietly spoken man who does not initiate conversation or ask for help if he needs it. The health care professional is concerned that John is reluctant to leave his bed and has become incontinent. There are concerns that John is becoming depressed by being in hospital. John's carers say that he has never been incontinent before. In discussion with John and his carers it is established that John is unclear where the toilets are because he says all the doors look the same.

A toilet symbol is put on the toilet doors nearest to John's bed.

Accessible information using photographs, diagrams, pictures and symbols are most useful when people have difficulty with written information and people have difficulty understanding spoken language. Some useful examples of symbols that may commonly be used in hospital settings can be found in 'The Hospital Communication Book'. A copy of this resource can be downloaded from: www.communicationpeople.co.uk/Hospital%20Book.htm.

Accessible information is particularly helpful for people who have memory difficulties. The patient can refer to the accessible information when they need to be reminded what has been explained to them. The document will ensure that the same information is reinforced each time the patient views it. When using photographs, diagrams, pictures or symbols it is important to ensure that the message is clear and unambiguous. What we perceive and the message that was implied can easily be misunderstood. (*Refer back to earlier section on perception.*)

The decision of which visual system to use to improve communication, be that photographs, diagrams, pictures or symbols, is dependent on the needs of the individual and in some circumstances, although this should not be the primary reason, the access to resources you have at the time. Whatever system is chosen it is important to review the images with the patient to ensure that the message the image represents has the relevant meaning.

Communication Case Study 9 – Use of images – Michelle

Michelle was planning to have cataract surgery. Michelle was able to express her needs verbally but her language comprehension as assessed by a speech and language therapist was around Age 6 Level. Michelle is extremely reactive to the body language and the intonation of the person talking to her. If she observed someone crying she would also cry. Staff noted that she would mimic your volume and tone, which often lead people to wrongly believe that she understood what she was being told.

During her pre-operative assessment her parents commented that Michelle always became very upset when she came into hospital, or had to have any tests or investigations. They were concerned that the more they attempted to reassure her, the more distressed she would become. It was noticeable that Michelle appeared to react to the nursing staff when they talked directly to her about what they were going to do, for example take her blood pressure.

Michelle liked to look at picture books. A book was made to help Michelle understand what would happen when she came into hospital. Michelle enjoyed talking through the book. This gave Michelle an understanding of the process of her admission.

On the day of admission Michelle brought her book with her to the hospital. The admitting nurse was able to talk to Michelle using her book, which she found less confronting than having the nurse talk directly to her. It helped Michelle to predict what would happen next, and she found directing the nurses to the book empowering and less like the nurse telling her what was going to happen.

How to develop an accessible treatment plan?

As previously explained, it is not always enough to tell a person verbally what is going to happen during their care and treatment. For individuals who have difficulty processing and retaining verbal information the use of pictures and/or symbols can be extremely effective. It is important, however, to consider the person's cognitive ability to process visual information when deciding whether to use drawings, pictures, symbols or letters and how these images should be presented.

The developmental process of relating images to words begins with naming objects. The person is able to relate the word cup to the object of a cup. The process then moves to photographic images, drawings, symbols and finally letters that make words. Therefore for most individuals the use of photographs to illustrate accessible information is generally more beneficial to aid understanding. However, the choice of images whether photographs, drawings or symbols must be very carefully considered to ensure that they accurately represent the information that needs to be given to the patient.

There are some very good examples of accessible information that have been devised by learning disability teams in partnership with hospitals and primary care providers. These are available from the valuing people website: www.valuingpeople.gov.uk.

An excerpt from an accessible information leaflet that could be used during a surgical admission is reproduced in Figure 3.5 with permission of the Shropshire County Primary Care Trust LD Community Nursing Service. This example shows the use of symbols/line drawings and photographs that illustrate the simple plain text. This document could be reproduced to be used by a number of individuals. In some circumstances, however, the needs of the individual may require you to produce an individualised document designed specifically to meet their communication needs. It is important that whatever you provide for the person, you ensure you check out before leaving it with them that they are able to understand the message you are trying to convey.

HELPING PEOPLE WITH LEARNING DISABILITIES TO MAKE CHOICES

Choice and control are key elements of person-centred planning and communication is often the way that choices are expressed. Communication difficulties can, therefore, present a barrier to making choices and health care professionals need to consider ways of overcoming these barriers and allow choices to be made. Accessible information is an extremely useful tool when

The Shrewsbury and Telford Hospital *NHS*
NHS Trust

South Staffordshire and Shropshire Healthcare *NHS*
NHS Foundation Trust

Welcome to The Day Surgery
At The Royal Shrewsbury Hospital

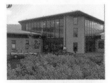

This is the Treatment Centre at the hospital where you will find the Day Surgery Unit.

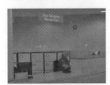

You need to go to the reception desk for Day Surgery.

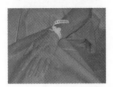

The person on the desk at Day Surgery will ask you to wear a bracelet that has your name on.

You will arrive in a room; it will look something like this.

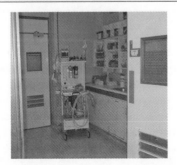

A doctor will place a small plastic tube into the area on your hand where the cream was applied then you will go to sleep for your operation.

Fig. 3.5   Example of accessible information leaflet. Reproduced with permission from Staffordshire and Shropshire PCT/A2A Network.

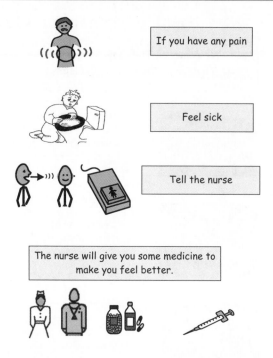

Fig. 3.5   (*Continued*)

helping people to make choices; however, not all people will need the use of additional resources to help them with decision making.

Reflective Learning Point:

Consider the choices you make every day. From the moment we wake in the morning we are constantly (usually unconscious of the fact that we are doing it) making decisions that will have impact on the day ahead. Some decisions are automatic because they are choices we have made many times in the past and they have become preferences, for example what we have for breakfast or whether to have tea or coffee. Other decisions made take a moment or two of conscious thought before making a choice, for example what to wear. Our choice in this case may be based on other external factor such as the activity for the day ahead or the weather outside.

The complexity of decision making can vary throughout the day from these more or less automatic decisions to having to decide whether to buy a new car or not, or whether to have a major operation that has been recommended by your surgeon.

Ferris-Taylor in Gates (1997) explains the complexity of the process of decision making and lists points to consider when supporting decision making.

- People need to be aware that choices are possible and available
- That there is an opportunity to make choices
- That the person has an awareness of or has experienced the choice being offered
- The person has an awareness of the consequences of making the choice

- Having an understanding of the financial constraints of making a choice or its impact on others
- Having the assertiveness to carry through the choice even if others disagree
- To have the skills to express the choice
- To be able to choose from a range of alternatives that is within memory and understanding capabilities

Advocacy and empowerment

Advocacy is essentially about speaking up, whether that is the person speaking for themselves (self-advocacy) or by another person or group of others speaking on behalf of the person. In health care situations there are times when we are faced with concerns of how to help the individual to express themselves.

The patient who presents unaccompanied may appear to be unable to give the relevant information or to fully understand the care or treatment plan recommended. In this situation it would be appropriate to ask if the patient has a person that would be able to act as an appropriate advocate for future consultations, by asking if there is a family member, friend or carer that they could contact to provide support. If they do not have such a person, it would be a good practice to recommend an advocate and obtain consent to refer for support from the local learning disability service.

Some patients will attend with a person who may be there to act as the person's advocate, for example a family member, carer or friend. This person may be a professional advocate such as a liaison nurse or independent mental capacity advocate. The health care professional needs to assess the status of the person accompanying the patient and confirm that the advocate is acting on the instruction of the patient.

Reflective Learning Point:

Susan attends the gynaecology outpatients department with her mother. Susan has cerebral palsy and a severe communication difficulty. Susan has come to discuss problems that she has been experiencing with menstruation on the request of her GP.

When called to the consulting room Susan's mother insists that she needs to be present during the consultation because 'Susan can't tell you what the problem is'. Susan looks worried. You ask if she wants her mother to come into the room. Susan looks at her mother and shrugs her shoulders.

What would you do?

Health care professionals are often faced with conflicts of interest when families and carers demand to be involved and informed. There are a number of issues to consider when deciding when to include another in the consultation and discussion about care and treatment; however, the crucial question is 'Does the patient consent to the advocate being in attendance?'

It is important to consider that many people with a learning disability have very little experience of making decisions for themselves as we discussed earlier in this chapter. For some individuals speaking up when they are accompanied by a person that they feel is in a position of authority can be extremely difficult and they may not be aware that they have the right to give their opinion. You may notice that the patient will look to the person supporting then when you ask a question. This is an indicator that the person is used to the carer speaking for them. It is important to redirect the question to the person to give them an opportunity to answer if they are able.

Friends, family and carers can both increase and restrict a person's ability to make choices. Jenkinson (1993) makes this example: 'The supporter may, when responding to choices made by a person with a learning disability, be resistant to supporting the decision if it is inconvenient or if it disrupts planned activities or established routines. Supporters may also exert more subtle influences by the way in which they define the problem and how questions are phrased, which will all influence a person's decision'. Jenkinson also notes that perceived social pressures can make the decision-maker highly resistant to a change of mind once a decision has been made and results in elevated levels of stress.

Goodley and Ramacharan (2005) suggest that a good advocate is likely to be able to distance themselves from the advocacy role. A good advocate will allow the patient to communicate with you to the best of their ability and will inform you of the best way to communicate with them. Knowing how to ensure an independent voice is a key task in the empowerment of the person with a learning disability to speak up and make choices. Empowering the person with a learning disability to express their problems, ideas, judgements and how they would like their needs to be met must be the priority goal for any advocate.

Parsloe and Stevenson (1992) define 'empowerment' as 'people having power to express their needs and to decide how these needs should be met'. A practical perspective by Dowson et al. (1998) defines empowerment in terms of individuals 'being enabled to have increased control over one's own life' and suggest that it involves the following features:

- Having information
- Being listened to
- Getting a response based on what has been said
- Sharing power with others who are appropriate to hold some of the power with the division of power clearly stated, protected and limited.

This has a direct impact on the health care professionals' relationship with a person with a learning disability. Empowerment does not mean giving all the power to the individual because by doing this Aldridge, in Jukes and Aldridge (2006, p. 31), explains that 'in empowering one individual there is a risk of disempowering others'. In real life, empowerment is usually represented by a balance of considering the needs of the individual and others, and understanding any limitations to choices.

The paternalistic approaches that used to be apparent in learning disability practice meant that the professional was considered to 'know best' and was in control of what happened to an individual. This was based on a rationale that people with learning disabilities were 'eternal children' and lacked the understanding and skills to take a directive part in their own lives. The development of self-advocacy groups such as People First has led to a change in approach. Aldridge, in Jukes and Aldridge (2006, p. 34), explained that 'the People First movement demonstrated that, with support, people with learning disabilities are capable of developing the skills to be self-directive and taking the lead in their own lives'.

Reflective Learning Point:

Health care professionals who use person-centred approaches act as an enabler for empowerment to take place.

COMMUNICATING WITH FAMILY AND CARERS

Promoting independence and empowering the patient must be the primary concern for the health care professional. However, family members and carers may also often feel that they are not consulted or listened to. Health care professionals need to be aware of their duty to maintain the right to confidentiality for the patient but understand that there are exceptions where it is appropriate to disclose information in the best interest of the patient who is unable to consent to the sharing of information.

Sir Jonathan Michaels (2008), in his report of the independent inquiry into access to health care for people with learning disabilities 'Healthcare for All', outlined some of the reports from carers regarding communication issues in health care. He reports that carers comment, 'Staff attitudes and values underpin their ability to communicate effectively with carers. Some communicate well. Others communicate very badly. Some do not communicate at all and seem to see carers as a nuisance'. The difficulties include:

- Failing to find a good balance between communicating to the person with a learning disability and communicating with the carer
- Failing to understand confidentiality issues (failing to share information, sometimes failing to respect a person's rights by saying too much)
- Failing to use plain language and/or pictures

He goes on to recommend the use of prior to admission information documents, to ensure continuity of knowledge, information, and standards of care, and to ensure all needs, including those relating to communication are acknowledged and an action plan in place to address those needs.

Even when you know the person with a learning disability can communicate independently, you should involve the carer in communication where necessary to ensure they do not feel excluded. The carer may sometimes be too embarrassed to offer information which they do not feel is important but may actually be vital to the care provided. The individual may not have told the carer everything about their health/symptoms and they may not be fully aware. In some situations you may find that the person does not want the carer to be involved in all aspects of their care and you will need to handle this sensitively.

You may be aware of the damning Health Service Ombudsman report 'Six Lives' (Parliamentary and Health Service Ombudsman 2009, p. 58) which investigated the premature deaths (in hospital) of 6 people with a learning disability. The report stated that the communication issue of passing information accurately between professionals and the family and then acting upon it was a key issue in the failings of the care for Mr. Ryan. 'Mr. Ryan himself was unable to communicate his needs. There was evidence that various professionals, including the community team and speech and language therapists, were very concerned about Mr. Ryan and tried to raise their concerns, particularly about nutrition, with the medical and nursing teams. But they could not make themselves heard and nothing happened to help Mr. Ryan. Nobody took any actions to feed him'. This highlights the importance of health care professionals communicating with family and carers. (*The ethical issues relating to this report are explored further in Chapter 6.*)

Family members and carers are an essential tool in the assessment of communication barriers and all current guidance highlights the need to listen to the people who know the person best. Although as we have discussed earlier there can be problems in that research suggests that carers often underestimate or overestimate the communication abilities of the person. However, when there are obvious communication issues, it is the carer who will be most likely to identify the non-verbal signals and the changes in behaviour that suggest the person is trying to communicate their needs.

CONCLUSION

This chapter highlights the importance of communication when working with people with a learning disability, and the specific skills that health care professionals need to develop in order to work effectively with this client group. Good communication is the basis of effective health care provision, and the value of developing a relationship and getting to know the individual demonstrates how this enables effective communication to take place.

Health care professionals need to develop competencies in identifying individual communication needs, and developing creative ideas for how to overcome these, using a range of tools to aid communication. Person-centred approaches provide a framework to do this on an individual basis, and also enable and support people to make choices.

Summary of Key Learning Points

The key learning points are:
- Effective communication using a range of key skills is essential for health care professionals when working with people with a learning disability.
- Developing relationships with people is an important part of the communication process – see the person and not the disability.
- More than half of people who have a learning disability have some level of communication difficulty.
- People with learning disabilities often feel that they are not given sufficient time to express themselves and communicate their needs.
- Poor listening skills have a significant part to play in diagnostic overshadowing.
- The Disability Discrimination Act 1995 requires all health care professionals to ensure that they must make adjustments to ensure that the patient is able to communicate effectively.
- Effective communication can be challenging but by making use of tools such as accessible information, communication can be enhanced.
- Find the best way to communicate:
  - Pay attention to facial expressions
  - Notice gestures and body language
  - Try using pictures or signing
- Keep information simple and brief and avoid using jargon.
- Communication with family and carers is also important, and they can be very helpful in establishing appropriate communication methods.

If you have concerns that you or your patient is having difficulties communicating there are others who can support you such as speech and language therapists, advocates and learning disability nurses.

Links to KSF Competencies – Chapter 3

KSF Dimension Core 1 – Communication

Level	Level descriptor
1	*Communicate with a range of people on day-to-day matters* For example, communicates with a limited range of people, reduces barriers to communication, accurately reports work activities, uses different forms of communication, communicates information only to people who need to know
2	*Communicate with a range of people on a range of matters* For example, communicates on a range of matters, effective use of communication skills, keeps accurate and complete records, manages barriers to effective communication, communication consistent with relevant legislation, helping others to communicate
3	*Develop and maintain communication with people about difficult matters and/or in difficult situations* For example, identifies a range of people involved in communication, communicates with people in a form consistent with their level of understanding, modifies communication to overcome barriers, provides feedback to others, seeking consent, sharing decision making, using communication aids, supporting people
4	*Develop and maintain communication with people on complex matters, issues and ideas and/or in complex situations* For example, identifies potential communication difficulties, encourages effective communication, anticipates barriers and takes action to improve communication, seeks out different styles and methods of communicating, explaining complex issues, contributing to decision making, sharing decision making, breaking bad news and supporting those receiving it

Reproduced under the terms of the Click-Use Licence.

REFERENCES

A2A – Access to Acute: A network for staff working with people with learning disabilities to support access to acute medical treatment (2009). Available at http://www.nnldn.org.uk/a2a./ Contact: rick.robson@sssft.nhs.uk.

Abudarham S and Hurd A (Eds) (2002) *Management of Communication Needs in People with a Learning Disability*. Whurr Publishers, London.

Bogdashina O (2005) *Communication Issues in Autism and Asperger Syndrome. Do We Speak the Same Language?* Jessica Kingsley Publishers, London.

British Medical Association Equal Opportunities Committee and Patient Liaison Group (2007) *Disability within Healthcare: The Role of Healthcare Professionals*. British Medical Association, London. Available at www.bma.org.uk.

Chambers S (2003) Use of non-verbal communication skills to improve nursing care. *British Journal of Nursing*, 12(14), 874–878.

Cogher L in Grant et al. (2005) *Learning Disability. A Life Cycle Approach to Valuing People*. Open University Press, Berkshire.

Cooper E (2009) Assessing contentment and distress. *Learning Disability Practice*, 12(1), 14–16.

Cumella S and Martin D (2000) *Secondary Healthcare for People with a Learning Disability*. A Report Completed for the Department of Health, Birmingham.

Disability Distress Assessment Tool (DisDat) (2004) Northgate Palliative Care Team and St. Oswald's Hospice. Contact: Dr. Claud Regnard 0191 285 0063 or e-mail on claudregnard@stoswaldsuk.org.

Department of Health (1995) *Disability Discrimination Act*. HMSO, London.

Department of Health (2005) *Mental Capacity Act*. HMSO, London.

Dowson S, Hersov E, Hersov J and Collins J (1998) *Action Empowerment: A Method of Self-Audit for Services to People with Learning Disabilities or Mental Health Support Needs*. National Tenants Resource Centre, Trafford.

Gates B (1997) *Learning Disabilities*. Churchill Livingstone, Edinburgh.

Goodley D and Ramacharan P in Grant et al. (2005) *Learning Disability. A Life Cycle Approach to Valuing People*. Open University Press, Berkshire.

Hannon L (2003) *Pre-Admission Assessment in Secondary Healthcare Services for People with Learning Disabilities*. Unpublished MSc Dissertation. University of Central Lancashire.

Jenkinson J (1993) Who shall decide? The relevance of theory and research to decision-making by people with intellectual disability. *Disability, Handicap and Society*, 8(4), 361–375.

Jukes M and Aldridge J (2006) *Person-Centred Practices. A Therapeutic Perspective*. Quay, London.

Kelly A (2000) *Working with Adults with a Learning Disability*. Wilmslow Press, Oxon.

Kevan F (2003) Challenging behaviour and communication difficulties. *British Journal of Learning Disabilities*, 31, 75–80.

Kurtz S, Silverman J, Benson J and Draper J (1998) *Teaching and Learning Communication Skills in Medicine*. Radcliffe Medical Press, Oxford.

Light J (1989) Toward a definition of communicative competence for individuals using augmentative and alternative communication systems. *Augmentative and Alternative Communication*, 5(2), 137–144.

Mehrabian A (1971) *Silent Messages*. Wadsworth, Belmont, CA.

Mencap (2002) *Am I Making Myself Clear? Mencap's Guidelines for Accessible Writing*. Mencap, London.

Michaels J (2008) *Healthcare for All. Report of the Independent Inquiry into Access to Healthcare for People with Learning Disabilities*. HMSO, London.

National Patient Safety Agency (2004) *Understanding the Patient Safety Issues for People with Learning Disabilities*. NPSA, London.

Nelson-Jones R (1993) *Practical Counselling and Helping Skills. How to Use the Lifestyle Helping Model*. Cassell, London.

NHS Scotland (2004) *Health Needs Assessment. People with a Learning Disability in Scotland*. NHSS, Glasgow, Scotland.

Parliamentary and Health Service Ombudsman (2009) *Six Lives: The Provision of Public Services to People with Learning Disabilities*. The Stationery Office, London.

Parsloe and Stevenson (1992) in Jukes M and Aldridge J (2006) *Person-Centred Practices. A Therapeutic Perspective* (p. 31). Quay, London.

Royal College of Nursing (RCN) (2006) *Meeting the Health Needs of People with Learning Disabilities: Guidance for Nursing Staff*. RCN, London.

Sandiford R (2004) I call it the rock and roll of nursing. *Nursing Times* 100(31), 28–29.

Silverman J, Kurtz S and Draper J (2005) *Skills for Communicating with Patients*, second edition. Radcliffe Publishing, Oxford.

Sowney M and Barr O (2007) The challenges for nurses communicating with and gaining valid consent from adults with intellectual disabilities within the accident and emergency care service. *Journal of Clinical Nursing* 16(9), 1678–1686.

Turnbull J (1999) Intuition in nursing relationships: the result of 'skills' or 'qualities'? *British Journal of Nursing*, 8(5), 11–24.

Tschudin V (1991) *Counselling Skills for Nurses*, third edition. Baillière Tindall, London.

4 Understanding Behaviour

INTRODUCTION

The evidence base shows that the anticipation of having to manage difficult behaviour is perhaps the one aspect of working with people with a learning disability that causes health care professionals the most anxiety and a fear of what to expect. In reality, a very small percentage of people with a learning disability exhibit what may be termed as 'challenging behaviour'.

Sir Jonathan Michaels (2008) identifies that around 15% of people with a learning disability display challenging behaviour, although these estimates vary depending on how challenging behaviour is defined.

Emerson et al. (2001) (cited in Grant et al. 2005) indicate that there are around 10–15% of people with a learning disability who present with challenging behaviour. Typical examples of challenging behaviour identified by Twist and Montgomery (cited in Grant et al. 2005) are:

- Verbal aggression
- Shouting
- Stripping
- Stealing
- Anal poking
- Self-injury
- Withdrawn from others
- Physical aggression
- Persistent screaming
- Inappropriate sexual behaviour
- Property damage
- Smearing faeces
- Disturbed sleep
- Non-compliance

Brittle (2004) documented that the unfamiliar environment of the acute hospital is likely to increase the levels of anxiety and distress for people with learning disabilities. Behaviours such as crying out, an inability to remain still, seeking comfort from a familiar object and rocking are often observed, along with other stereotypical behaviours that the person may adopt to provide comfort, as a coping mechanism or as a means of self-stimulation.

This chapter intends to reassure health care professionals that working with behavioural issues is not as difficult as they often expect. The aim is that by developing a better understanding

General Hospital Care for People with Learning Disabilities, First Edition by Lynn Hannon and Julie Clift
© 2011 Blackwell Publishing Ltd

of the individual and the possible function of the behaviour, the health care professional can develop a clearer insight into what the behaviour may mean and its purpose for the individual.

Simple behavioural approaches are introduced that health care professionals can use to respond to behaviour in health care situations, and ideas for psychological approaches are also included. A detailed section devoted to the assessment of pain is included as this is often a reason for behavioural symptoms being displayed. Risk assessment and the use of restraint and physical interventions are also explored, with good practice guidance included.

Whilst a small number of people who exhibit some very difficult behaviour may need specialist assessment and intervention, the majority of people and their behavioural needs can be managed within the normal environment with a small amount of preparation.

WHAT DO WE MEAN WHEN WE SAY A PERSON DISPLAYS CHALLENGING BEHAVIOUR?

Definitions

Over the years there have been a number of definitions and descriptions given to people with learning disabilities. Some of these terms have led to very negative stereotyping of learning disability, and in particular to the perception that people with learning disabilities are physically aggressive towards others and their environment, and are unable to act appropriately in the community. Even in today's supposed more enlightened times, with consideration of political correctness in the way that we view disability, these negative perceptions such as imbecile, sub-human, idiot, mad and eternal child continue to be used.

People with learning disabilities are like the rest of us in that there are times when aspects of our personality and behaviour may be found to be irritating by those around us. For most of the time people either ignore the behaviour, chose to avoid us, or may tell us when we are behaving in a way they find objectionable. For some people with learning disabilities there are times when the behaviour they display is more extreme than the norm, and people find this difficult to accept and avoid being with the person therefore leading to social isolation.

Definition:

Challenging behaviour is the term generally used to describe behaviour that significantly affects the relationships the person has with others and has an impact on their daily living.

There may be a multitude of possible needs that the person is trying to communicate through their behaviour. Trying to translate these behaviours can be challenging even to the most experienced. Thorough investigation of the situation by asking those who know the person well and comprehensive observation of the behaviour can lead to a greater understanding of the patient's experience.

Challenging behaviour may manifest in response to a number of factors including:

- Relationship and emotional needs: A way of expressing feelings, fear, anger and disappointment.
- Life events: In response to dealing with past experiences that may have been difficult or abusive.

- Response to physical need such as pain or discomfort.
- Changes to the environment or going to places that are unfamiliar. The demands of the hospital environment can be disturbing for some individuals. The sights, smells sounds and equipment can be overstimulating and evoke fear and anxiety. This can been extremely distressing for some individuals and if the distress that the environment is causing is not identified, it can easily escalate into severe challenging behaviour leading to significant self-harm.
- Mental health issues: Studies investigating the prevalence of psychiatric problems in adults with a learning disability and challenging behaviour found an increase in psychiatric problems and self-injurious behaviours appear related to increased levels of anxiety (Moss et al. 2000).

However, these terms are often how people have tried to describe what they observe when they experience a person with a learning disability who is displaying behavioural distress. Gates et al. (2000) explain that terms such as 'behaviour problems', 'disturbed behaviour' and more recently 'challenging behaviour' as introduced by Blundell and Allen (1987), all attempt to categorise what is in general terms 'behavioural distress'.

Behavioural distress

According to Gates et al. (2000), there is no common agreement regarding the definition of this phenomenon. They cite Emerson et al. (1988) and Emerson's definition of challenging behaviour, 'Severe challenging behaviour refers to behaviours of such an intensity, frequency or duration that the physical safety of the person or others is likely to be placed in serious jeopardy, or behaviour that is likely to seriously limit or deny access to and use of ordinary community facilities'.

By using the term 'challenging' there is an assumption that the behaviour displayed may in some way proceed to cause harm to the individual, or more commonly the belief that the behaviour may cause harm to others. What this definition does highlight is the result that challenging behaviour can limit the person's access to community services. In particular, for people with learning disabilities, this can affect their access to health care.

The term 'behavioural distress' as defined by Gates et al. (2000) is more helpful in that it transfers the focus from what the outcome of the behaviour my result in, to what the behaviour is communicating. By establishing the cause of the distress we are able to gain an insight into how the person is experiencing their world and how we can adapt the environment to reduce the incidence of the behaviour occurring. It must be acknowledged however that this often takes hours of 'functional analysis' (the thorough assessment of the person including the environment) and the development of strategies to prevent injury or reduce the negative impact of the behaviour which can be effective but requires an investment in time and effort. (*See later section on 'Assessment and Observation of Behaviour' for more information about functional analysis.*)

Self-injurious behaviour

The term 'self-injurious behaviour' refers to any activity in which an individual inflicts harm or injury to him or herself. Self-injury can take many different forms, including:

- Head banging (on floors, walls or other surfaces)
- Hand or arm biting
- Eye gouging
- Hitting areas of the body and face

- Skin picking, scratching or pinching
- Inserting objects into the body
- Hair pulling

The reasons a person engages in self-injurious behaviours are varied, and will often involve a complex interaction of physical and social factors. Eye poking that may have started as a form of sensory stimulation may develop into a way to gain attention.

There may be a connection between types of self-injury and tic disorders and compulsions. Clements and Zarkowska (2000) suggest that high stress levels are believed to increase the frequency of these uncontrolled movements.

Lyon and Pimor (2004) highlight that in some instances there is a strongly suggested link between organic factors and challenging behaviour in particular self-injurious behaviours. Lip biting is associated with Lesch–Nyhan and Cornelia de Lange syndromes; knuckle biting with Lesch–Nyhan syndrome; and Hypomelanosis of Ito (including wrist biting) finger and toe nail picking and head banging with Smith–Magentis syndrome; and temper tantrums and voracious eating in Prader–Willi syndrome.

These behaviours are not necessarily provoked by feeling of anxiety or used necessarily as a means to communicate need, but may be problematic behaviours for health care professionals in their attempt to assess and provide care and treatment. In cases where self-injurious behaviour is a known behaviour for the individual it is essential that the health care provider consults family or carers in the best management of these behaviours.

It is essential to respond quickly to incidents of self-injury even if the behaviour serves the function of gaining attention from others. It is never appropriate to ignore severe self-injurious behaviour.

Try to limit verbal comments, speak calmly and keep facial expressions neutral to avoid inadvertently reinforcing the behaviour. If the individual is finding it difficult to cope with demands being placed on them, cut back on the demands being placed on them or stop the activity entirely. Come back to the activity again later when the person is feeling calmer. Re-directing the individual to another activity and/or gently guiding the hand or head away from the self-injury. It may be necessary to place a barrier, such as a pillow, between the individual and the object that is causing harm. Where the self-injurious behaviour places the individual at serious risk of harm it may be appropriate to explore the use of physical restraint. (*For guidance on the use of restraint see later section in this chapter.*)

Challenging behaviour, sometimes displayed in the form of self-injury, may be the person's way of exhibiting that they are experiencing abuse. It is widely accepted that adults with learning disabilities are victims of abuse and neglect. They are at increased risk as a result of their vulnerability due to the lack of insight into what constitutes abuse and an inability to communicate that they are experiencing abuse. Health care professionals need to be aware of the potential for abuse being a cause of challenging behaviour and consider this within their assessment. (*See section on safeguarding children and vulnerable adults in Chapter 6 for further information on abuse.*)

WHAT COULD DIFFERENT BEHAVIOURS MEAN?

It is important when making judgements to think about what the person is trying to communicate by their behaviours. For people with a learning disability, a hospital admission can be particularly stressful, resulting in behaviour that is not usual for them. A lack of understanding of social rules can cause confusion and may lead to behaviour that appears inappropriate to others. People with autistic spectrum disorders may find particular difficulties in interacting with unfamiliar people and may engage in particular kinds of behaviour in order to avoid or limit social contact.

Reflective Learning Point:

You are sitting on the beach watching the waves splashing onto the shore. A young man is swimming in the sea and you notice that he is trying to gain your attention. Is he waving or is he drowning?

What aspect of this man's behaviour would tell you that he was in distress?

Functional analysis

There may be a multitude of possible needs that the person is trying to communicate through their behaviour. Trying to translate these behaviours can be challenging even to the most experienced. Thorough investigation of the situation by asking those who know the person well and comprehensive observation of the behaviour can lead to a greater understanding of the patient's experience. This is known as 'functional analysis'. May (2005, p. 10) described this as 'Gathering together behavioural clues and developing a hypothesis or theory to explain why a behaviour is occurring'.

The aim of functional analysis is to identify the behaviours that are challenging, explore the frequency, duration and intensity of the behaviour, and assessment of all aspects of the environment, including how the person communicates, lifestyle, relationships and any other relevant information. (*See later section on 'Assessment and Observation of Behaviour' for more information about functional analysis.*)

Causes of challenging behaviour

Herbert Lovett, a psychologist with a particular interest in learning disability and challenging behaviour, states that in his experience 'extreme behaviour often comes from not feeling listened to'. He says that as helpers we often do not respond to the messages the person is trying to covey because, 'if people communicate without words we cannot hear them' (Lovett 1996).

Ephraim (cited in Hewitt 2001), also a psychologist, explains that people with learning disabilities use behaviour to communicate their needs, in particular when they feel pain, feel unheard or unloved. He describes this as 'exotic communication'.

It is thought that there are a number of causes of challenging behaviour. McDonnell 1995 (cited in Kelly 2000) gave nine common causes that he believes are instantly recognisable to those who work with people with learning disabilities:

1. Being unable to communicate
2. Being in pain
3. Changes in routine
4. Being confused
5. Changes in medication
6. Inactivity

7. Attention-seeking behaviour
8. Environmental effects
9. Delusional thoughts

If we consider this list of possible causes of challenging behaviour in acute service settings, any of these could be a possible reason for the behaviour.

Reflective Learning Point:

If you saw someone banging their arm against their head what do you think could be a potential cause for this behaviour?

Some possible causes to consider could be tinnitus, earache, headache, toothache, being unable to communicate, frustration, boredom, feeling frightened or unsure about what was happening to them, or feeling that no one was paying attention to them. Identifying the cause helps the health care professional to understand the function of the behaviour.

Behaviour that challenges typically falls into one or more of the following categories:

• Sensory stimulation
• Gaining attention
• Tangible reinforcement
• Escaping from demands

Fear and anxiety are often the main cause when people with a learning disability refuse or are non-compliant with treatment. When supporting someone with a learning disability who is anxious about treatment the person may display avoidance type behaviours that can be observed as:

• Asking to go home
• Asking to wait until later
• Running away
• Smacking you
• Refusing to engage with you, for example looking away when being spoken to
• Changing the subject, for example asking when it is time for lunch

These are responses that are characterised by the perception of harm, pain or lack of control, which may come from a lack of understanding of what is happening to them. It is important that interactions with the person, if based on a cognitive approach, should be truthful and positive and dispel the myth that treatment will be painful and distressing, although it may be necessary to discuss that there may be an element of discomfort.

Important areas to explore

• Is this a normal behaviour for the person? – What is already known about the person and what is the understanding of the function of that behaviour?

- Personal characteristics and usual indicators of mood: For example, bangs hand on table when hungry, noises they make.
- Physical needs: Has the person's sleep pattern been disturbed? Are they hungry?
- Expressions when there are changes in routine: For example, normally would be able to give verbal response but due to the anxiety of talking to a stranger is unable to respond to questioning.

Reflective Learning Point:

John has severe learning disabilities and visual impairment. He has come into hospital for an outpatient's appointment escorted by his carer. He has been seated in the waiting area where he has been waiting for 5 minutes. John starts to walk up and down in the waiting area.

- What do you think could be the possible reasons for this behaviour?
- What would you do/say to John?

It is important when making judgements to think about what the person is trying to communicate by their behaviours. This understanding of what the behaviour might mean can only be really developed through experiential learning. Working with a wide range of people with learning disabilities and gaining a better understanding of their needs enables health care professionals to develop a more confident approach in dealing with behavioural issues.

Reflective Learning Point:

Think about how easily you can interpret the behaviour of a person you know well. They often do not need to communicate verbally to tell you that something is wrong you just know it is.

- What are the clues you pick up on that make you aware that something is wrong?

Diagnostic overshadowing

Why is it so important to carefully assess what the behaviour is telling you? 'Diagnostic overshadowing' was highlighted in the Disability Rights Commission (DRC; 2006) formal investigation *Equal Treatment: Closing the Gap*. It highlighted failings in access to, and delivery of appropriate treatment in primary care for people with learning disabilities. The report suggested that there was a failure for staff to listen or understand, and a tendency to attribute heath problems to the persons' learning disability, and for illness to be overlooked as a result of this.

Michaels (2008) [1.2.3] explained that 'Witnesses reported that the phenomenon is widespread and is particularly problematic in palliative care or when someone with a learning disability is in pain and can only communicate distress through behaviour (such as screaming or biting) that staff find challenging and/or difficult to interpret'. The inquiry heard many examples of this problem and he continued to report that [5.2] 'Although diagnostic overshadowing may occur in relation to other groups (such as older people, or people with mental health problems), our witnesses argue that learning disabilities represent a special case'.

The key recommendation made to overcome this is to ensure that both undergraduate and post-graduate clinical training includes mandatory training in learning disabilities. The expectation is that better trained staff are more aware of specific health needs, have a more positive approach to people with a learning disability, and are less likely to stereotype people.

Clinical decisions checklist

Northgate Palliative Care Team and St. Oswald's Hospice (2004) use a clinical decisions checklist to identify possible reasons for behavioural changes that are not usual for the person and could indicate a physical cause. This may be particularly helpful with people who cannot communicate verbally. The checklist is illustrated in Table 4.1.

This checklist represents one tool that you may find useful and is included as an example of a method of understanding behaviour. Of course the specific cause of the behaviour may be something else that is not covered on this checklist, but even if the answer to everything here is 'NO', it will help you to eliminate a number of potential causes and point the focus to another area.

Table 4.1 Clinical decisions checklist

Clinical decisions checklist Is the new sign or behaviour?	YES	NO
• **Repeated rapidly?** *Consider* pleuritic pain (in time with breathing) *Consider* colic (comes and goes every few minutes) *Consider:* repetitive movement due to boredom or fear		
• **Associated with breathing?** *Consider:* infection, COPD, pleural effusion, tumour		
• **Worsened or precipitated by movement?** *Consider:* movement-related pains		
• **Related to eating?** *Consider:* food refusal through illness, fear or depression *Consider:* food refusal because of swallowing problems *Consider:* upper GI problems (oral hygiene, peptic ulcer, dyspepsia) or abdominal problems		
• **Related to a specific situation?** *Consider:* frightening or painful situations		
• **Associated with vomiting?** *Consider:* causes of nausea and vomiting		
• **Associated with elimination (urine or faecal)?** *Consider:* urinary problems (infection, retention) *Consider:* GI problems (diarrhoea, constipation)		
• **Present in a normally comfortable position or situation?** *Consider:* anxiety, depression, pains at rest (e.g. colic, neuralgia), infection, nausea		

Source: Clinical decision checklist from DisDAT. Northumberland Tyne & Wear NHS Trust and St. Oswald's Hospice (2008).

HOW HOSPITAL ADMISSION CAN AFFECT INDIVIDUAL BEHAVIOUR AND WAYS OF OVERCOMING THIS

People with a learning disability are often vulnerable and frightened when admitted to hospital. We have identified that some people with a learning disability may find being in the unfamiliar environment of the acute hospital distressing, and that this distress may present itself in behaviours that are challenging for those attempting to assess and give treatment. Prevention of stress and anxiety will reduce the likelihood of reactive behaviours developing into behaviours that challenge and the need for the use of physical interventions.

Important components in a supportive environment for effective management of people who may display challenging behaviour are:

- *Relationships*: Positive calm and flexible approach of staff towards the person, with attention to staff who have a particular rapport with the person providing care.
- *Communication*: Promoting the autonomy of the person by providing information in a way that the person is able to understand. It is important to be flexible but too much negotiation can provoke more anxiety and therefore the likelihood of the person refusing to be compliant with or agree to the treatment proposed. It can be helpful to reduce the level of demands when a person is upset or agitated and therefore it may be necessary to put off discussion or decision making until the person is less stressed.
- *Environment*: Assessment of the physical environment and removal of any stress provoking stimulus, such as too much noise, equipment, or just giving the person some personal space can help to reduce stress.
- *Medication*: Ensure that any anti-psychotic medication continues to be prescribed during the admission and that its effectiveness is reviewed.
- *Use of alternative therapies*: For some individuals the use of alternative therapies such as massage and relaxation techniques can prove to be valuable, especially if this is something they have previously been introduced to and associate it with a positive activity.

The following case study illustrates a real example where a communication misunderstanding caused a behavioural response.

Understanding Behaviour Case Study 1 – Mary

Mary was admitted to hospital for cholecystectomy. Mary had Prader–Willi syndrome and moderate learning disabilities. The main clinical features of Prader–Willi syndrome are:

- Excessive appetite often leading to obesity
- Low muscle tone
- Emotional instability
- Immature physical development
- Learning disabilities (sometimes very mild)

Mary was recovering well from her surgery when she developed a pulmonary embolism and required further treatment. Due to no visible or palpable access to peripheral veins the doctors had been having difficulty inserting a cannula.

Mary's mother was concerned because the ward staff frequently asked her to stay with Mary on the ward because when she left Mary would cry and throw herself on the floor. Mary's mother also believed that Mary was hallucinating because she was saying unusual things such as 'they are talking about me' and 'I am not a beast'. Mary's mother felt that this was not usual for Mary and the doctor suggested that she may have an infection that could be causing her to hallucinate.

During a period when Mary was calm she was asked what was causing her to be distressed. Mary said that she wanted to leave the hospital because the doctors were mean to her. When asked what the staff had done to make her feel this way she said that the doctors had said she was 'a beast'. After much thought as to what this might mean, when asked if she meant 'obese' she said yes. She said that she could hear the doctors talking about her when they stood at the desk. It was explained to Mary that 'obese' is a medical term to describe her condition but that it would not be used if she would prefer them not to.

Mary was reassured that the doctors would not use this term again and staff were instructed to be more careful when discussing patients away from the bed. This reassured Mary and the admission was completed without further problems.

The staff involved with this case had accepted that because of her learning disability the behaviour she was displaying was a response to her not wanting to be on her own in hospital. An assumption was made that because she was saying things that are not usual for her that there was an underlying mental health problem. By listening to Mary and clearly observing her behavioural distress it became clear that it was her language difficulties and her inability to engage with someone who understood what she was trying to express that was the cause of her distress.

This also illustrates that it is important to establish that the patient understands the terms that are used. For Mary being described as 'obese' was not familiar to her and she had converted this to a word she did understand. It is clear from this example that being described as a 'beast' would be distressing for anyone. (*For more information regarding managing communication difficulties see Chapter 3.*)

Understanding Behaviour Case Study 2 – Rose

Rose is a 51-year-old woman with a severe learning disability. She has limited communication skills, though can understand most things said to her. She exhibits a number of difficult behaviours including, screaming, hitting people and throwing objects. Rose needs full help with personal care and also with general mobility. She has been in hospital before and was admitted on this occasion for surgery.

She was supported during her admission by a paid carer from the private residential home she lives in, and was visited by her community LD nurse. The carer had supported Rose on previous admissions. The community nurse has 19 years of nursing experience and has known Rose for 8 years. The hospital staff working with Rose was a qualified nurse, and midwife, with 15 years of experience. She had worked with people with a learning disability in hospital before.

Following completion of a pre-admission assessment (see Chapter 2) it was decided Rose would use a single room to provide her with personal space, more room for carers and to minimise potential for disruption on the ward. The carer felt that [7.19] 'If she was in a room of her own she would have less opportunity to go and upset other patients'. However, on the second day of her stay she had to be moved onto a four-bed bay due to the needs of another patient. The hospital staff explained about Rose to other patients on the bay, and they were very accepting of her.

The hospital staff maintained regular contact and did not leave the carer to provide all her care. Hospital staff said her first thought when someone with a learning disability was being admitted was [8.186] 'How are we going to cope?' but [8.193] 'We coped very well with Rose. We didn't have any problems'.

Communication and behaviour problems are known to influence the process of health care for people with a learning disability. Hospital staff were aware of the potential problems and planned for them, supported by the carer and community nurse. Surgery was completed as planned, and the admission was seen as successful by all stakeholders (Hannon 2003).

(Reference numbers in brackets refer to interview transcripts from the research project.)

This case study demonstrates that even the most difficult behaviours can be coped with in the hospital setting if detailed pre-admission assessment and person-centred care planning take place. General hospital services need to be flexible and responsive to individual need, making reasonable adjustments to ensure that people access the health care required to meet their needs.

Some ideas for ways of overcoming the impact of a hospital admission on behaviour can include:

- Pre-admission visits
- Bring familiar belongings into hospital
- Involve the person in preparing for the hospital stay as much as possible, for example packing their own bag, choosing toiletries to take with them
- Preparing communication tools (if appropriate) to explain procedures
- Get support from a carer or someone who knows the person well to identify any potential behavioural needs in advance
- Spend time settling the person into the hospital environment
- Adapt the environment to meet the needs of the individual
- Maintain usual routines where possible
- Ensure a range of activities are available to keep the person occupied
- Have a flexible approach to timekeeping to avoid putting additional pressure on the person
- Maintain usual sleep pattern
- Use of simple behavioural or psychological approaches (see later in this chapter)

HOW TO RESPOND TO BEHAVIOUR IN HEALTH CARE SITUATIONS

Whilst the use of behavioural approaches is a highly skilled area of expertise, there are a number of straightforward approaches that can be used by general hospital staff without any specific training in behavioural approaches. The attitude of health care professionals towards the person with a learning disability is an important aspect of working with behavioural needs as this influences your perception of what is happening and the reasons behind it.

Lovett (1996) reminds us that 'whilst we often enlist the support and advice of families and carers to help us decide how to address and change behaviour, how often do we think about how to change our own behaviour in response to the person'? If we always react in the same way we will generally always get the same response.

Fear of the unexpected and a lack of training in learning disabilities means that many health care professionals have a negative attitude and lack confidence in dealing with behavioural needs. This has also led to a perception that this is a particularly difficult aspect of working with people with a learning disability. As highlighted in the evidence base in Chapter 1 – difficult situations do tend to stick in the mind and this needs to be balanced out with positive experiences gained from working with people with a learning disability. Initial fears are often changed in the light of experience, leading to a more positive attitude.

In reality, a small number of people will present with challenging behaviour of such a degree that additional support will be required. Very little environmental change is needed. Most people are able to mix with other patients and blend into the usual ward surroundings and activities. Whilst the choice of a single room is appropriate for some people, there is no need to put people there as a matter of course.

How to describe behaviour

It is often how the behaviour is described that causes a negative response from those observing or being informed about the person and their needs. For example:

1. John – 'Be careful he's a biter'.
2. Elizabeth – 'You need to keep an eye on her she often does a runner'.

This type of description of the behaviour of people with learning disabilities is commonly heard, and can create anxiety and suggest that the person is problematic. This description also creates an image of the person that influences your perception and can affect the way you respond to the person when you first meet them.

By changing the language we use to describe the behaviour we can be more helpful in informing what support the person needs.

1. John – 'John does not like to be in unfamiliar places. He does not like to be touched by people he does not know. When John becomes distressed in these situations he sometimes makes attempts to bite to communicate that he wants you to keep away from him'.
2. Elizabeth – 'It is important to supervise Elizabeth in unfamiliar places because when she is anxious she will attempt to leave the environment very quickly'.

You can see how changing the way that the behaviour is described presents a completely different image of the person, and also gives you clues as to interventions that will be needed to support them during their stay in hospital.

Assessment and observation of behaviour

As outlined earlier in this chapter, a *'functional analysis'* is needed in order to understand or explain why a behaviour is occurring. It is particularly important that when observing behaviour we describe behaviour accurately, and that we ensure that this agrees with the descriptions of others. This will ensure that the final description we make of the behaviour observed, is truly reflected in how the behaviour is described, and is understandable to all those who are involved in the management of the behaviour.

May (2005, p. 10) suggests that 'In order to complete such an analysis, we need to gather information about what happens before, during and after a behavioural incident, and understand any relevant background factors that may be contributing to the behavioural difficulty. From this information, we are then able to establish whether or not there are any patterns and can form a hypothesis as to why the behaviour is occurring'.

It is vital to identify the potential reason for the behaviour in order to identify the best response to use to minimise the likelihood of the behaviour occurring. Failure to base interventions of how to respond to behaviour, on the specific cause of that behaviour, is likely to result in ineffective and unnecessarily restrictive practice.

Behaviour that challenges typically falls into one or more of the following four categories:

- Sensory stimulation, for example head banging, eye poking, pain relief
- Gaining attention
- Tangible reinforcement, for example to get access to desired items or activity
- Escaping or avoiding demands

Therefore, a functional analysis of behaviour must explore these four functions alongside the environmental factors when making an assessment of the function of any behaviour.

To determine the function of the behaviour there are three methods for obtaining the information.

1. Interviews with relevant others
2. The use of rating scales
3. Manipulating different environmental events to see how this affects the behaviour and direct observation of the behaviour utilising 'antecedent behaviour consequence' charts (ABC charts)

Method 3 – ABC – is considered the more reliable method for assessment.
May (2005, p. 10) defines ABC as:

- *Antecedent*: What occurs immediately before the behavioural outburst
- *Behaviour*: A description of what actually happened or what the behaviour 'looked like'
- *Consequence*: What happened immediately after the behaviour

It can also be a good idea to keep track of where and when the behaviour occurred to assist in identifying any patterns.

Table 4.2 demonstrates a simple ABC chart format for recording behaviour.

From the information obtained from these briefly documented observations it can be established that the person uses a similar pattern of behaviour which is crying and head banging. You will notice that removing the source used for head banging does not always reduce the behaviour. The individual will often find an alternative source for self-injury if the preferred source is removed. However, it is sensible to remove any objects that are likely to cause significant injury to the person and to make attempts to protect the person from physical injury.

Table 4.2   ABC chart

Date and time	Antecedent What was happening before the behaviour commenced?	Behaviour What did the person do, for how long?	Consequence What happened after the event?
11/05/2009 11.00 am	Carer was helping to change the bed Carer left to go for a cup of tea	Crying out and periodically banging forehead on the side of the bedside locker for 10 minutes	Distracted from banging with book and cup of tea
12/05/2009 11.15 am	Doctor's visit – blood taken	Crying and rocking on the floor by the bed Banging head on the bedside locker for 10 minutes	Assisted back into bed by carer, bedside locker removed, crying continued for 10 minutes
14/05/2009 11.10 am	Resting in bed	Banging head on the table, rocking and crying for 5 minutes	Walked to the dayroom to watch the television
14/05/2009 11.25 am	Sitting in the dayroom with nurse	Crying and banging head with hand for 5 minutes	Distracted from banging with puzzle book, continued to cry
15/05/2009 16.35 pm	Returning from the bathroom	Crying out and banging head with hand, rocking and banging hand on table, for 15 minutes	Family visiting, crying and banging continued for 5 minutes

You will also note that the time of the incidents is fairly consistent. You may consider what happens at this time each day:

- Is the ward noisier than usual?
- What would the person normally be doing at this time if they were at home?

Reflective Learning Point:

- Look on the ABC chart at the antecedent for each occurrence of behaviour and identify what you think could be possible reasons for this person's behaviour?
(Use the four functions of behaviour outlined earlier which may help you to identify possible reasons for this patient's crying and head banging.)

You may observe particular behaviours during the hospital admission that will require detailed observation and assessment. It is important to consider, when a patient with learning disabilities is presenting with behaviour that is challenging, who is the most appropriate professional to provide this assessment. Some learning disability nurses are appropriately qualified to support with this type of assessment. However, there may be situations that require more specialist assessment from a clinical psychologist or behavioural therapist. Your local learning disability team will be able to help in making arrangements for a specialist assessment if required.

Behavioural approaches

When addressing any behavioural problem it is important to select just one or two areas to focus on at a time. This reduces the potential for the individual to become confused about what your interventions are dealing with. Behavioural change takes time and you would usually choose to work first on the behaviours that are of most concern, or are having the biggest impact on the individual's life.

The use of behavioural approaches is a highly skilled intervention and care must be taken to ensure that effective approaches are used that are appropriate to achieve the outcome you are aiming for. This section introduces some of the more commonly used approaches that may be useful for health care professionals, though an experienced behaviour therapist will have many more options to consider.

Reinforcement

The use of reinforcement to encourage desirable behaviour and modify a person's behaviour is well recognised. May (2005) explains that 'Positive reinforcement is the strengthening of a particular behaviour by following it with something desirable. Positive reinforcement should be used as a component in almost all behavioural interventions, to facilitate the development of new skills, encourage appropriate behaviour and enhance self-esteem'.

She continues to state that reinforcers can take a number of different forms including:

- Favourite foods – edibles
- Toys or objects – tangibles
- Activities
- Praise or social reinforcement
- Sensory-based reinforcers

You may already be familiar with the use of preferred foods, especially sweets to coerce a child to cooperate with a blood test for example, or the use of star/sticker reward charts and good behaviour certificates.

> Reflective Learning Point:
>
> Think how you feel yourself when someone gives you praise for something. It will almost always encourage you to repeat that behaviour and makes you feel good.

The decision to use behavioural approaches should not be made lightly or without the knowledge of how to assess the need, and the skill to devise and implement a strategy that is appropriate to the person's needs. Basic principles that must be applied when using reinforcement in health care situations are:

- That all health care professionals and carers involved in the implementation of the reinforcement strategy are consistent, sensitive, committed and motivated. All those involved in the use of the reinforcement must follow the reinforcement schedule set out in the care plan. *Reinforcement is effective only if used consistently*. Any concerns from members of the health care team or by the carers must be established before the use of reinforcement commences.

- That the reinforcer is outside the person's normal routine. This is where food and drink should not be used. It can be tempting to use a pending meal or drink to motivate a person to comply with a procedure. Promising that if they comply they will receive a drink or their meal is inappropriate.
- Reinforcement must not in any way compromise the rights and integrity of the person. At no time should the reinforcer be used if, by not complying with the desired behaviour, the persons attempt to communicate is ignored.

Reinforcement works best when it is provided *immediately* after the desired behaviour has occurred. The following case study demonstrates the use of a token reward scheme to reinforce a desired behaviour.

Understanding Behaviour Case Study 3 – Reinforcers

It has been decided to use a reinforcer to encourage Paul to participate in his physiotherapy. Paul has been reluctant to participate in his physiotherapy after a fall when he fractured his hip because he feels pain when he mobilises. He is unable to understand that this pain is normal and that he needs to mobilise to aid his recovery.

The physiotherapist discusses the need for the mobilisation therapy to his care workers. It is agreed that Paul will receive a token that he can exchange for items from the hospital shop when he participates in his physiotherapy.

Care must be taken not to misunderstand Paul's signs if he does not comply with the physiotherapy. It may be that Paul has pain, feels too tired or is unwell.

The following case studies are real-life examples of the use of reinforcement:

---

1. Three-year-old Mohammed constantly climbs on to people's laps rather than sitting on his own chair. His parents provide verbal praise and a tickle each time he sits on his chair independently.
2. Max's hand-flapping behaviour interferes with his ability to concentrate on his school-work. His teacher recognises that the hand-flapping may provide important sensory input for Max, so has devised a programme whereby reinforcement is provided for reduced hand-flapping during periods of desk work.
3. Jane displays a range of challenging types of behaviour during lunchtimes at school. The members of staff have decided that reducing aggressive behaviour towards other students is a priority and so give Jane positive reinforcement for those periods of time when there is no aggressive behaviour, even though she is still exhibiting other types of undesirable behaviour.

May (2005, p. 10)

Prompting

Different levels of prompting can be used to help individuals learn new skills or encourage them to complete a task or an activity.

Prompts can take the form of:

- Physical prompts – for example, holding someone's arm to guide them
- Gestural prompts – for example, using gestures to demonstrate what you want someone to do
- Verbal prompts – for example, telling someone how to do something
- Environmental prompts – for example, a picture on the wall that shows someone how to do something

Prompts can be used successfully with positive reinforcers to promote behavioural change and skill development.

Reflective Learning Point:

Think about prompts or positive reinforcers that you have received that helped or encouraged you to complete something at work.

- What kind of prompts were they?
- Why did they work for you?

Redirection

This may be a useful intervention to use when you are trying to deal with a person who is distressed about a health intervention that you need to perform.

May (2005, p. 10) highlights that 'Redirecting an individual's attention to a preferred topic of conversation or activity can be an extremely effective way of preventing escalation and defusing a difficult situation'. She continues to suggest that 'It can be helpful to have a range of calming and distracting activities lined up so that they are ready to use if the individual starts to become agitated'.

This is something that you can prepare for if the potential need is identified during pre-admission assessment. Identifying this early will give you time to develop strategies and activities that you can use to redirect the person's attention to a different activity. Relaxation techniques are particularly useful when helping people cope with distress and can help to refocus the person away from the activity that is causing them to become anxious.

In general, behavioural approaches are intended to provide strategies to develop a planned response to a behavioural incident or outburst. Table 4.3 summarises some key points that you may find helpful.

Psychological approaches

Psychological approaches such as '*systematic desensitisation*' and '*cognitive behaviour therapy*' used in the mainstream are found to be well supported for overcoming individual fears/anxiety and barriers to care. Gordon et al. (1998) suggest that 'cognitively impaired persons will rarely benefit from behavioural approaches', however, the benefits of using these approaches effectively with this client group have now been demonstrated.

Table 4.3 Behavioural approaches summary

Possible triggers	Strategies to try
• Changes to routine • Medical issues, such as pain or illness • Frustration at communication difficulties • Stressful social occasions • Sensory overload	• Environmental modifications • Use of alternative or augmentative communication strategies (see Chapter 3) • Redirection to relaxing, neutral activities • Removal of trigger (or individual) from environment
Possible cues of distress	**Strategies to try**
• Facial expressions • Bodily movements or gestures • Repetitive behaviour • Yelling, shouting	• Responding calmly and clearly • Removing demands • Reinforcing calm behaviour • Redirecting to a neutral activity • Removing the individual or others from the environment
Possible types of behaviour	**Strategies to try**
• Aggression towards others • Injuring themselves • Destroying property • Tantrums	• Responding calmly and clearly • Ensuring that the environment is safe • Removing yourself and others from the environment to ensure safety, and continue to observe individual from a distance • Get extra help if needed • Providing the minimal response required until individual begins to calm down
Possible behaviour	**Strategies to try**
• The behaviour may be reducing intensity or have ceased, but the person may still be agitated or distressed	• Give the individual space to calm down • Redirect individual to a neutral activity and give praise for appropriate behaviour • Reinforce calm behaviour • Wait until individual has calmed completely before raising issue or making demands

Adapted from May (2005). Reproduced with kind permission from the National Autistic Society.

Systematic desensitisation

Prangell and Green (2008) discuss the debate that psychological approaches such as systematic desensitisation *are* useful in helping people with learning disabilities. They highlight that the evidence to suggest that these approaches are not useful in helping people with learning disabilities is inconclusive. They suggest that the adaptation of cognitive-behavioural approaches can be successful in their study of 'dental anxiety'.

In the authors' experience the skilled application of a number of psychological/cognitive approaches can be extremely useful and effective in overcoming barriers to care.

Understanding Behaviour Case Study 4 – Systematic Desensitisation/Gradual Exposure to Treatment

Colin was known to have an inguinal hernia that needed surgery. Colin has epilepsy and severe learning disabilities. It was agreed that Colin could not consent to the procedure and that surgery would be in his best interest. However, Colin's support staff did not feel that they would be able to support Colin at the hospital as they had encountered many problems in the past. At the pre-operative assessment Colin had refused to go into the consulting room and had become distressed when the nurse tried to talk to him. Sedation had been tried previously but had failed and Colin had been more distressed than ever.

Colin's staff worked on a gradual desensitisation programme to introduce him to the hospital. The care staff brought Colin to the hospital where he met with the liaison nurse. These visits increased and led to him paying a visit to the day surgery waiting area to meet with the nursing staff.

Colin gradually gained his confidence enough to sit in the day surgery waiting area and talk with the nursing staff for them to be happy that an admission day could be planned. Along with a well-planned admission Colin was able to have his surgery without the need for medication or restraint.

This case study demonstrates the importance of taking time to get the intervention right and also how this positive experience means that Colin is more likely to receive future treatment successfully based on this.

Cognitive behaviour therapy

Challenging automatic thoughts – It is common for all of us to expect the worst when we face a situation we have not been in before and anticipate that it either is going to be painful or may cause distress. Automatic thoughts are just such ideas that automatically come to mind when a particular situation occurs.

They are characterised by a vicious cycle of automatic negative thinking. By using a 'thought stopping statement' such as 'if I cannot stand the pain I will ask the nurse to stop' or 'this may hurt me but it will only be for a few seconds' can change the negative thought into a more helpful empowering thought. Then find something to do that takes the concentration, interest, and focus away from the old negative, vicious-cycle thoughts.

Many people are able to identify a need to do this for themselves. However, those patients who present with anxiety around health care procedures may benefit from a more structured approach known as cognitive-behavioural therapy (CBT).

CBT is a short-term talking treatment that has a highly practical approach to problem solving. It aims to change patterns of thinking or behaviour that are behind people's difficulties, and so change the way they feel. Some people with learning disabilities need help to identify how to challenge what these thoughts are as they may not be able to identify their own strategy.

Self-affirming statements can help to reassure an individual when they are feeling anxious or that they are not coping, for example, I'm OK', 'I'm doing well', 'I can do this'. By encouraging these statements, repeating and reaffirming the statement with the person can be reassuring and helps them to feel in control.

The following case study demonstrates how CBT approaches can avoid the use of restraint or physical interventions.

Understanding Behaviour Case Study 5 – Regaining Control – Stop Signals

Bill needed dental treatment but was anxious because of what he described as 'rough' treatment by dentists in the past. Bill's negative thoughts were identified as 'It'll hurt', 'I can't cope', 'I don't know what will happen'.

Bill was introduced to a number of coping strategies to help him manage these automatic thought about dental treatment. Bill received information regarding his treatment in an accessible format known as his 'book'.

Statements like 'I know what's going to happen – I can check my book' and 'If I want them to stop I can ask them to stop' were suggested for him to use when he was feeling anxious prior to and during the procedure. He was encouraged to use statements like 'Didn't I do well' after the treatment. Bill was also taught some basic relaxation techniques to use during the treatment. A stop signal was agreed which for Bill was that he would raise his hand when he wanted the treatment to stop.

The evaluation of this process was that the combination of these techniques was successful for Bill and helped him to receive the dental treatment he required.

The following case study highlights how using tools that empower the person to control their environment can be beneficial in reducing the level of anxiety they experience.

Understanding Behaviour Case Study 6 – Relaxation Techniques

Clare had been admitted after collapsing at home. She was found to have a low haemoglobin level due to problematic bleeding haemorrhoids. Clare needed a blood transfusion but was refusing to allow the nurse to start her transfusion.

Clare had been given accessible information to understand why she needed the transfusion and was assessed as having capacity to decide not to have the treatment. Clare discussed her anxiety about the transfusion. She related the experience that her father who had died of leukaemia 2 years previously had had a number of transfusions. She understood why transfusions were necessary but she could not detach the fear she felt when her father was transfused with the need for the procedure herself. The thought made her panic and not be able to allow the nurse to continue.

We talked about how we could support her through this anxiety and identified that she had used relaxation techniques in the past to help her with anxiety. We tried hand massage which Clare said she found relaxing. During the hand massage Clare was encouraged to imagine positive things that she wanted to do in the future. Clare then agreed to try this approach while the nurse set up her transfusion. Clare did not want to be told that the process had started so the nurse quietly proceeded while Clare was relaxing.

Clare became aware that the process had started, and although acknowledged that she felt anxious, she did not want the process to stop. Clare completed her transfusion and was able to go on to have further transfusions in the future.

This case study demonstrates the importance of establishing a calm and reassuring atmosphere when carrying out health care procedures for people who are highly anxious. Basic breathing and relaxation techniques have been found to be beneficial for reducing anxiety and providing coping skills for people with learning disabilities, enabling necessary health care interventions to be completed.

Solution-focused approaches

As health care professionals we are often faced with difficult situations that we need to overcome. We spend time considering how to support patients to achieve the required outcome, sometimes preparing complex assessments and behavioural programmes, only for the patient to refuse to comply with the treatment.

By being problem focused, for example 'How are we going to get the treatment completed because the patient will not co-operate?', we can become frustrated by our lack of achievement and we can often begin a cycle of negativity for the patient who may feel even more anxiety and lack of control in the situation. If we shift our problem-solving approach to one of looking at the skills of the individual and how they feel they can achieve the outcome we can develop a more positive alternative strategy. This type of approach is known as solution-focused therapy.

The solution-focused brief therapy model was devised by Steve de Shazer in the 1970s and is a collaborative approach that encourages people to talk about preferred futures rather than the pathology of the problem. This approach is utilised by therapists working with people who are experiencing a number of difficulties to help them develop strategies to overcome issues such as addiction and behavioural problems.

A solution-focused approach is a way of working that encourages the patient to move forward rather than remain stuck in a problem or in behaviour. The approach encourages the patient to consider times when, for instance, the problem behaviour has not been displayed or the individual has dealt with the difficulty differently.

When we experience difficulties, we often get lost in the thoughts of failure but when we investigate the exceptions to this, reflect on our strengths, ask questions about our achievements – we can regain some experience of any small success and build on this. We can help patients to identify and attend to their skills, abilities and external resources (e.g. social networks). This process not only helps the patient to see themselves as a competent individual, but also aims to help the patient identify new ways of bringing these resources to bear upon the presenting problem.

One of the basic principles of a solution-based approach is that the *patient knows best*. By allowing the patient to lead the process one of the most important aspects of a successful intervention can be achieved, that being trust in the health care professional and their desire to help the process.

When questioning the patient, encourage them to think differently about themselves and the difficulty they are experiencing. This may include looking at times when the patient faced similar experiences that caused them anxiety in the past and how they overcame their fear, and particularly focuses on the achievement of being able to cope and that they achieved the outcome they wanted. For some people with a learning disability this may be a difficult process and they may rely on a family member or carer to remember these occasions.

This model for care planning differs greatly from our usual problem-solving approach as the health care professional acts as a conduit for change rather than acting as a prescriptive expert.

Understanding Behaviour Case Study 7 – Solution-Based Approaches

Donna needs to have dental treatment under general anaesthetic. Donna has moderate learning disabilities and is able to consent to the procedure. Although Donna fully understands the need for her procedure, and because of the level of pain she is experiencing wants to have her surgery soon, she has an intense fear of having an anaesthetic.

Donna worked with the pre-assessment nurse and the learning disability liaison nurse to try to establish how they could help Donna overcome her fear of the anaesthetic room. The usual approaches were tried such as pre-visits to the hospital and accessible information. She had attended for an admission but refused to go into the anaesthetic room at the last minute.

Donna described how she felt able to cope when she went to the blood room because the nurses were quick and rarely asked any questions. Donna felt that keeping the talking to a minimum helped her to remain focused on getting the task done. She felt that people asking her the same questions over again and checking out that she was OK caused her to start worrying about 'not being OK'.

Donna felt that by health care staff keeping their verbal interactions to a minimum and by acting promptly she would be able to control her anxiety. She also felt that she was able to control her feelings better if she could focus on issues unrelated to the procedure. Donna said that she listens to music when she is feeling anxious so she decided she wanted to be able to take her personal music player with her into the anaesthetic room.

Prior to the day of admission Donna and the pre-operative nurse reviewed the procedure she would have to ensure she was fully informed of what would happen when she goes to theatre. They completed an admission care plan that outlined her wishes with regard to how she would like the health care staff to communicate with her.

On the day of the admission all the staff that would be working with Donna that day were briefed on her wishes for them to keep any verbal interaction to a minimum, and that she did not want them to talk about what was going to happen. The focus of interactions was light-hearted and Donna enjoyed having a joke with the health care assistant allocated to support her.

When the time came to go into the anaesthetic room Donna began to show signs that she was feeling anxious. She was reminded to put on her music and was given lots of verbal encouragement that she was coping well. While the anaesthetist prepared to cannulate Donna he talked about the music she was listening to as a distraction. The theatre nurses joked with Donna about the anaesthetist preferring to listen to Tom Jones than her choice of Westlife.

Donna was soon in theatre and her operation completed.

This case study demonstrates that focusing on a positive solution helped Donna to feel in control of the process of her admission to hospital.

Restraint and physical intervention

The use of restraint and/or physical interventions can create ethical dilemmas for the health care professional. The main consideration is to balance the need for the person to receive the health care they need with protection and respect of their rights as an individual.

People with learning disabilities have the same legal protection as any other person. Therefore, any restrictive practice that places a constraint on a person's liberty must always be professionally but more importantly legally justified. Decisions about preventing the person or others coming to harm are often based on the concern for protecting the person from coming into harm without breaking the law, and ensuring that we are maintaining our duty of care.

The circumstances that lead up to the use of physical intervention are often after an episode of agitation or aggression. Staff may be tempted to use a physical intervention in the first instance when an alternative strategy may be more appropriate.

The law in England and Wales allows all citizens to live without interference from others. There are three forms of interference that can be found in both civil and criminal law, those being:

1. *False imprisonment*: For example, confinement in a room, being prevented from leaving a room, being restrained in a chair.
2. *Assault*: Direct physical or verbal intention to harm (use of threatening words). 'Any act – and not a mere omission to act – by which a person intentionally or recklessly causes another to apprehend immediate unlawful violence. ... The act must be accompanied by hostile intent'. Richardson et al. (2003) cited in BILD (2008).
3. *Battery*: Similar to assault but actual physical force must take place. This could be any type of touching even to the clothing. There is no need to prove that harm or pain has been caused.

There are other less common but relevant criminal offences contained in the Offences Against the Persons Act (1861) including:

- Assault occasioning actual bodily harm
- Malicious wounding or inflicting grievous bodily harm
- Manslaughter
- Murder

Other relevant legislation:

- Mental Health Act 1983 (Department of Health 1983)
- Human Rights Act 1998 (The Stationery Office 1998)
- Mental Capacity Act 2005 (Department of Health 2004)

The law in Scotland is similar but with some substantial differences.

- Assault – physical contact must occur
- Culpable recklessness – the unintentional causing of harm as a result of accident or recklessness
- Homicide
- Culpable homicide – the equivalent of manslaughter

In Scotland, criminal law has a specific legal acknowledgement for the use of restraint where there is evidence of danger or risk of personal injury; this is termed 'restrain a lunatic'.

Other relevant legislation and guidance can be obtained from:

- Mental Health (Care and Treatment) (Scotland) Act 2003
- Adults with Incapacity (Scotland) Act 2000

Book Reference: British Institute of Learning Disabilities (2008) *Physical Interventions: A Policy Framework* (second edition) can provide a more detailed application of the law and the use of physical intervention.

BILD (2002) and (2008) recommends two key principles for policy to ensure the protection of individuals within the law:

1. Any restrictive physical intervention should be consistent with the legal obligations and responsibilities of care agencies and their staff and the rights and protection afforded to people with learning disabilities under the law.
2. Working within the 'legal framework', services are responsible for the provision of care, including restrictive physical interventions, which are in the person's best interests.

The Mental Capacity Act 2005 provides health care professionals with a framework to ensure that whenever we are making decisions on behalf of a person who lacks capacity that those decisions are made in the person's 'best interests'. If restraint is to be used the health care professional must have a reasonable belief that the person lacks capacity and that the act is necessary to prevent or protect the person from coming to harm.

Conditions that justify restraint are:

- The person taking action must reasonably believe that it is necessary to do an act that requires restraint in order to prevent harm to the person who lacks capacity.
- The act must be a proportionate response in both the degree and duration of the restraint to the likelihood of the person suffering from harm and the seriousness of that harm.

The health care professional must be clear and unbiased in their reasoning for the justification of the intervention. Restraint must not be used simply to enable staff to do something more quickly or easily.

Typical situations where restraint may be considered are:

- When the patient requires urgent medical treatment in the emergency department and is un-cooperative with the person attempting to deliver treatment.
- The patient tries to leave the ward or department without supervision and is believed to be at risk.
- The patient requires urgent tests or investigations to establish cause of significant symptoms, for example endoscopy.
- In pre-operative preparation (anaesthetic departments).
- To prevent the patient from getting out of bed or the chair due to risk of falling.

Reflective Learning Point:

* How would you prevent a patient from leaving your department if you thought they were at risk if they left?
* How would you prevent a person from falling out of bed?
* Do you have guidance you could follow to assist your decision-making process?
* Have you been trained in the safe use of restraint/physical intervention techniques?

Physical interventions are known to present risks to both the patient and staff, particularly when the restraint is unplanned. There have been documented deaths of people with learning disabilities dying as a result of inappropriately applied restraint. Murphy et al. 2002 (cited in BILD 2008) argue that 'poor practice would be less likely to occur if there is a clear policy framework for the use of physical intervention'.

In circumstances where it is identified that restraint is/may be required it is essential that the intervention is risk assessed. There are three central components to any risk assessment:

1. Significance of the outcome
2. Actions to reduce the risk
3. Recording and review

The following case study demonstrates the process of risk assessment and making decisions in the best interests of the patient.

Understanding Behaviour Case Study 8 – Restraint

Tom has severe learning disabilities and autism. He is a very large man, 1.88 cm (6 ft 2 inches) tall and 142.5 kg (22 stones) in weight. Tom requires treatment under general anaesthetic. Tom does not like to be touched by anyone including his carers.

Normally a very gentle man he has never required any level of physical intervention before except when attempts were made to take blood because of concerns that he may have developed diabetes. These attempts have failed despite desensitisation methods being employed. The decision is taken to plan an admission to hospital. As part of the pre-operative assessment the issue of restraint to manage Tom in the anaesthetic department is risk assessed.

Due to Tom's physical size it is decided that a physical intervention would not be a safe option for him or the staff supporting him. In discussion with the anaesthetist it is decided that he will be administered medication to sedate him prior to being taken to theatre as the least restrictive option.

The use of any form of restraint or physical intervention should be considered as a 'last resort' response and should only be implemented following specific training in safe use of the intervention. When a physical intervention has been used that was not planned, for example in the emergency department, it is necessary to document the action taken and the reasons for that action in the patient's case file. The incident should be reported as with any other clinical incident in accordance with Reporting of Injuries, Disease and Dangerous Occurrences Regulations 1995. (*See also Chapter 5 for further information about consent.*)

THE USE OF BEHAVIOURAL INDICATORS IN THE ASSESSMENT OF PAIN

As outlined earlier, this chapter has explored the meaning or function of behaviour and it has been identified that pain could be a contributing factor in the change of behaviour in the patient. The Royal College of Nursing Institute (1999) states that 'The goal of pain assessment is to ensure that effective procedures and processes are instituted to prevent or minimise pain'. The accepted gold standard for the assessment of pain is to ask the patient and to be guided by what they tell you. There is evidence of the effectiveness of this strategy and, according to Wood (September 2008), assessment of pain is 'the fifth vital sign in patient assessment' and a crucial component of pain management.

When assessing patients with a learning disability, it cannot always be determined by the use of self-reporting measures such as analogue pain scales which are the usual method and considered the most accurate guide on the patient's pain experience. There is also a need to assess cognitive ability as reduced cognitive ability leads to an individual being less likely to be able to self-report and a difficulty in localising pain. There is also evidence to suggest that some people with a learning disability do not present in the expected manner to pain, even though the pain may be acute, and abnormal behaviour may occur as a reaction to pain.

We have to consider that some people with learning disabilities would be unable to verbally articulate their pain experience and therefore the health care professional must establish another strategy for establishing the level of pain experienced by the patient. It is estimated that 50% of people with a learning disability will have a significant communication difficulty and therefore there is a need to have other tools for pain assessment, other than the gold standard of patient reporting, to aid the assessment of the patient.

Pain assessment in people with learning disabilities requires a skilled approach. A combination approach amalgamating observation and verbal assessment is recommended by Lebus et al. (2003)), and Foley and McClutcheon (2004) state that 'It appears that the best pain assessment is skilled clinical assessment with familiarity and understanding of the patient'.

In the Health Service Ombudsman's report (2009, p. 38) it was identified that one of the cases investigated was subject to suffering from a fractured thighbone. The report states that Mark's pain management was inadequate, 'His urgent need for pain relief was not met and assessment and planning for ongoing pain management was not of a reasonable standard'. Mark is described as moaning and in obvious distress, unable to sleep or settle. He was admitted to hospital where it took 3 days for him to be assessed by the pain team. The full details of the case are not documented but it would suggest that Mark's behaviour would clearly identify that he was experiencing some pain and that this should have been responded to immediately. [Mark's case study was originally described in the Mencap (2007, p. 11) report, *Death by Indifference*, which presented the stories of six people with a learning disability who had died in whilst hospital care.]

Understanding non-verbal communication and behavioural indicators could be the key to effective pain management for people who are unable to self-report.

This is important even for people who have good communication skills as they may not always be able to express what they are feeling. A vital clue to what the person is trying to communicate is the ability to identify the changes in the person's non-verbal signals and observable behaviour. To be able to achieve this the health care professional needs to know what are the norms for the patient and this information can be solicited from the people who know them best, the family or carers.

Table 4.4 Behavioural observations caregivers use to determine pain in non-verbal, cognitively impaired individuals

Vocal: Moaning, whining, whimpering (fairly soft), crying (moderately loud), screaming/yelling (very loud), a specific sound or vocalisation for pain, a word, cry, type of laugh.

Eating/Sleeping: Eats less, not interested in food, increase in sleep/decrease in sleep.

Social/Personality: Not cooperating, cranky, irritable, unhappy, less interaction, withdrawn, seeks comfort or physical closeness, difficult to distract, not able to satisfy or pacify.

Facial expression of pain: Crying, grimace, furrowed brow, change in eyes, including eyes tight closed, eyes open wide, eyes as if frowning, turn down of mouth, not smiling, lips pucker up, tight pout or quiver, clenches teeth, grinds teeth, chews, thrusts tongue.

Activity: Not moving, less active, quiet, jumping around, agitated, fidgety.

Body/Limbs: Floppy, stiff, spastic, tense, rigid, gestures to or touches part of body that hurts, projects, favours, or guards part of the body that hurts, flinches or moves body part away, sensitive to touch, moves body in a specific way to show pain (e.g. head back, arms down, curls up).

Physiological: Shivering, changes in colour, pallor, sweating, perspiring, tears, sharp intake of breath, gasping, breath holding.

Source: McGrath et al. (1998), cited in Davis and Evans (2001). Reproduced from the *British Journal of Nursing* with kind permission of Mark Allen Publishing.

Profoundly learning disabled people often use more than verbalisation to communicate. Facial expression, body movement and vocalisations which may be the norm for the person could be misinterpreted as signs of distress by the carer who is not familiar to them. Studies have shown that behaviours that are not usual could be an indicator, for example the 'quiet inactivity' as described by Chivall 2001 (cited in Foley and McClutcheon 2004).

Astor (2001) explained that 'Pain that goes unnoticed and not treated can lead to the patient feeling frustrated and distressed leading to the person displaying self injurious behaviour'.

Table 4.4 identifies a number of behavioural observations that could be used in pain assessment. (*See also Chapter 3 for further information about non-verbal communication.*)

Pain assessment tools

The use of specific pain assessment tools is familiar to many health care professionals but, as outlined earlier, these often rely on a self-reporting of pain (site, degree of pain etc.) which some people with a learning disability may not be able to do. The following tools are examples of appropriate tools that could be used for pain assessment in people with a learning disability.

The paediatric pain profile

The *Paediatric Pain Profile* (2003) was devised by University College, London/Institute of Child Health and the Royal College of Nursing Institute, to help in assessment and monitoring of pain in children with severe neurological impairments, especially those who are unable to communicate through speech. The authors state that 'Such impairments mean that the children are dependent on their carers for interpretation of their signs of pain. These signs may include changes in the child's movement and posture, in vocalisation and in facial expression'. The *Paediatric Pain Profile* is designed to pick up those behaviours which have been shown in a series of studies to be the most important indicators of pain.

The profile documents a description of the child under normal circumstances and highlights indicators of pain to aid communicating the child's experience to professionals in the diagnosis of illness and to monitor the intensity and duration of pain.

We hope you will find the tool useful. Copies can be obtained through the following link: www.ppprofile.org.uk.

If you have any questions or comments about the tool, do feel free to contact: Dr Anne Hunt, Research Fellow, RCN Institute, Radcliffe Infirmary, Oxford OX2 6HE, Tel: 01865 224392, Email: anne.hunt@rcn.org.uk

Disability Distress Assessment Tool

'Distress may be silent, but it is never hidden'

The Disability Distress Assessment Tool (DisDAT 2008) designed by the Northumberland Tyne & Wear NHS Trust and St. Oswald's Hospice is intended to help identify distress cues in people who because of cognitive impairment or physical illness have severely limited communication. The DisDAT is designed to describe a person's usual content cues content, thus enabling distress cues to be identified more clearly. It documents what many staff have done instinctively for many years thus providing a record against which subtle changes can be compared. This information can be transferred with the client or patient to any environment (Fig. 4.1).

The process of completing the DisDAT is as follows:

1. Observing the client when content and when distressed.
2. Observing the context in which distress is occurring.
3. Use the clinical decision distress checklist.
4. Treat or manage the likeliest cause of the distress.
5. Monitor how the distress changes over time.
6. The goal is a reduction in the number or severity of distress signs and behaviours.

This tool relies on observed signs and behaviours to identify distress in people of any age with severe communication difficulties of any causes and has features which help with monitoring and assessing the cause of the distress. For a full-size version of the tool in colour, for more information about DisDAT and to obtain the assessment and monitoring documentation, see www.disdat.co.uk.

FURTHER READING

Regnard C, Reynolds J, Watson B, Matthews D, Gibson L, Clarke C. Understanding distress in people with severe communication difficulties: developing and assessing the Disability Distress Assessment Tool (DisDAT). *J Intellect Disability Res* 2007; 51(4): 277–292.

Disability
Distress Assessment Tool

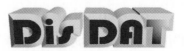

Northgate Palliative Care Team and St. Oswald's Hospice

Client's name:

DoB: Gender:

Unit/ward: NHS No:

Your name: Date completed:

Names of others who helped complete this form:

INFORMATION AND INSTRUCTIONS ARE ON THE BACK PAGE

Facial appearance when CONTENT

Face

Tongue/jaw

Eyes

Facial appearance when DISTRESSED

Face

Tongue/jaw

Eyes

Vocal signs when CONTENT

Sounds

Speech

Vocal signs when DISTRESSED

Sounds

Speech

Habits and mannerisms when CONTENT

Habits

Mannerisms

Comfortable distance

Habits and mannerisms when DISTRESSED

Habits

Mannerisms

Comfortable distance

Posture & observations when CONTENT

Posture

Observations

Posture & observations when DISTRESSED

Posture

Observations

Context of distress and communication/action which helps ease distress

(You can record eithera specific episode, using dates, or just describe what usually causes this person to be distressed)

Date	Context of distress	Actions that can alleviate distress

Fig. 4.1   Disability distress assessment tool. Reproduced from Regnard et al. (2007).

Disability
Distress Assessment Tool

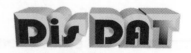

Please take some time to think about and observe your client's appearance and behaviours when they are both content and distressed, and describe these cues in the spaces given. We have listed words in each section to help you to describe your client or patient. You can circle the word(s) that best describes the content and distress cues in each category and, if possible, give a fuller description in the spaces given. Your descriptions will paint a clearer picture of your client or patient.

COMMUNICATION LEVEL*

This person is unable to show likes or dislikes	☐ Level 0
This person is able to show that they like or don't like something	☐ Level 1
This person is able to show that they want more, or have had enough of something	☐ Level 2
This person is able to ask for and anticipate their like or dislike of something	☐ Level 3
This person is able to communicate detail, qualify, specify and/or indicate opinions	☐ Level 4

* This is adapted from the Kidderminster Curriculum for Children and Adults with Profound Multiple Learning Difficulty (Jones, 1994, National Portage Association).

FACIAL SIGNS

Appearance

Information / instructions	Appearance when content	Appearance when distressed
(Ring) the word that best describes the facial appearance	Passive Laugh Smile Frown Grimace Startled Frightened Other:	Passive Laugh Smile Frown Grimace Startled Frightened Other:

Jaw movement

Information / instructions	Movement when content	Movement when distressed
(Ring) the word that best describes the jaw movement	Slack Grinding Biting Other:	Slack Grinding Biting Other:

Appearance of eyes

Information / instructions	Appearance when content	Appearance when distressed
(Ring) the word that best describes the appearance	Good eye contact Little eye contact Avoiding eye contact Closed eyes Staring Sleepy eyes 'Smiling' Winking Vacant Tears Dilated pupils Other:	Good eye contact Little eye contact Avoiding eye contact Closed eyes Staring Sleepy eyes 'Smiling' Winking Vacant Tears Dilated pupils Other:

SKIN APPEARANCE

Information / instructions	Appearance when content	Appearance when distressed
(Ring) the word that best describes the appearance	Normal Pale Flushed Sweaty Clammy Other:	Normal Pale Flushed Sweaty Clammy Other:

Fig. 4.1   (Continued)

VOCAL SOUNDS (NB. The sounds that a person makes are not always linked to their feelings)

Information / instructions	Sounds when content	Sounds when distressed
(Ring) the word that best describes the sounds *Write down* commonly used sounds (write it as it sounds; 'tizz', 'eeiow', 'tetetetete'):	**Volume**: high medium low **Pitch**: high medium low **Duration**: short intermittent long **Description of sound / vocalisation**: Cry out Wail Scream laugh Groan / moan shout Gurgle Other:	**Volume**: high medium low **Pitch**: high medium low **Duration**: short intermittent long **Description of sound / vocalisation**: Cry out Wail Scream laugh Groan / moan shout Gurgle Other:

SPEECH

Information / instructions	Words when content	Words when distressed
Write down commonly used words and phrases. If no words are spoken, write NONE		
(Ring) the words which best describe the speech	Clear Stutters Slurred Unclear Muttering Fast Slow Loud Soft Whisper Other:	Clear Stutters Slurred Unclear Muttering Fast Slow Loud Soft Whisper Other:

HABITS & MANNERISMS

Information / instructions	Habits and mannerisms when content	Habits and mannerisms when distressed
Write down the habit or mannerism. E.G. "Rocks when sitting"		
Write down any special comforters, possessions or toys this person prefers.		
Please (Ring) the statement which best describes how comfortable this person is with other people being physically close by	Close with strangers Close only if known No one allowed close Withdraws if touched	Close with strangers Close only if known No one allowed close Withdraws if touched

BODY POSTURE

Information / instructions	Posture when content	Posture when distressed
(Ring) the word that best describes how this person sits and stands.	Normal Rigid Floppy Jerky Slumped Restless Tense Still Able to adjust position Leans to side Poor head control Gait: Normal / Abnormal Other:	Normal Rigid Floppy Jerky Slumped Restless Tense Still Able to adjust position Leans to side Poor head control Gait: Normal / Abnormal Other:

BODY OBSERVATIONS

Information / instructions	Observations when content	Observations when distressed
Describe the pulse, breathing, sleep, appetite and usual eating pattern, eg. eats very quickly, takes a long time with main course, eats puddings quickly, "picky".	Pulse: Breathing: Sleep: Appetite: Eating pattern:	Pulse: Breathing: Sleep: Appetite: Eating pattern:

Fig. 4.1 (*Continued*)

Information and Instructions

Whenever we communicate face-to-face we don't just use words or writing. *Our face* reveals emotions such as joy, contentment, fear, anger and sadness. *Our voice* can provide clues through its tone and quality. *Hands* are used extensively to emphasise, illustrate or hide our feelings. *Posture* shows our feelings and can indicate whether we are being defensive, trusting or frightened.

DisDAT is

Intended to help identify distress cues in people who because of cognitive impairment or physical illness have severely limited communication.
Designed to describe a person's usual content cues content, thus enabling distress cues to be identified more clearly.
NOT a scoring tool. It documents what many staff have done instinctively for many years thus providing a record against which subtle changes can be compared. This information can be transferred with the client or patient to any environment.
Only the first step. Once distress has been identified the usual clinical decisions have to be made by professionals.
Meant to help you and your client or patient. It gives you more confidence in the observation skills you already have which in turn will help you improve the care of your client or patient.

WHAT TO DO

1. **Observe the client** when content and when distressed- document this on the inside pages. *Anyone* who cares for the patient can do this.
2. **Observe the context** in which distress is occurring.
3. **Use the clinical decision distress checklist** on this page to assess the possible cause.
4. **Treat or manage** the likeliest cause of the distress.
5. **The monitoring sheet** is a separate sheet which may help if you want to see how the distress changes over time.
6. **The goal** is a reduction the number or severity of distress signs and behaviours.

Remember

- Most information comes from the whole team in partnership with the family.
- The assessment form need not be completed all at once and may take a period of time.
- Reassessment is essential as the needs of the client or patient may change due to improvement or deterioration.
- Distress can be emotional, physical or psychological. What is a minor issue for one person can be major to another.
- If signs are recognised early then suitable interventions can be put in place to avoid a crisis.
-

Clinical decision distress checklist
Use this to help decide the cause of the distress

Is the new sign or behaviour?

- Repeated rapidly?
Consider pleuritic pain (in time with breathing)
Consider colic (comes and goes every few minutes)
Consider: repetitive movement due to boredom or fear.

- Associated with breathing?
Consider: infection, COPD, pleural effusion, tumour

- Worsened or precipitated by movement?
Consider: movement-related pains

- Related to eating?
Consider: food refusal through illness, fear or depression
Consider: food refusal because of swallowing problems
Consider: upper GI problems (oral hygiene, peptic ulcer, dyspepsia) or abdominal problems.

- Related to a specific situation?
Consider: frightening or painful situations.

- Associated with vomiting?
Consider: causes of nausea and vomiting.

- Associated with elimination (urine or faecal)?
Consider: urinary problems (infection, retention)
Consider: GI problems (diarrhoea, constipation)
- Present in a normally comfortable position or situation?
Consider: pains at rest, infection, nausea.

If you require any help or further information regarding DisDAT please contact:
Lynn Gibson 01670 394 260
Dorothy Matthews 01670 394 179
Dr. Claud Regnard 0191 285 0063 or e-mail on
claudregnard@stoswaldsuk.org

Further reading
Regnard C, Matthews D, Gibson L, Clarke C, Watson B. Difficulties in identifying distress and its causes in people with severe communication problems. *International Journal of Palliative Nursing*, 2003, 9(3): 173–6.

**Distress may be silent,
but it is never hidden**

Fig. 4.1 *(Continued)*

When using any tool of this type when attempting to interpret behaviour as an expression of communication it is important to remember that:

- Most information comes from the whole team in partnership with the family.
- The assessment form need not be completed all at once and may take a period of time.
- Reassessment is essential as the needs of the client or patient may change due to improvement or deterioration.
- Distress can be emotional, physical or psychological. What is a minor issue for one person can be major to another.

Having an assessment document like the tools suggested means that the health care professional is armed with the information they require to act promptly when pain is suspected. If signs of pain are recognised early then suitable interventions can be put in place to avoid a crisis.

Not all patients will present with this level of assessment available. The clinical decisions check list (see earlier in this chapter) can be a useful starting point along with a pain assessment tool that was originally devised for elderly people with dementia by the Royal College of Physicians (RCP 2007).

The Abbey Pain Scale

The Abbey Pain Scale is included in the 'National Guideline for the assessment of pain in older people' developed by the RCP, British Geriatrics Society and British Pain Society (2007). The scale is a tool for the measurement of pain in people with dementia and not only incorporates the behavioural and communication indicators of pain but also includes physical and physiological changes for the individual.

The guideline is 'an instrument designed to assist in the assessment of pain in residents who are unable to clearly articulate their needs' and the authors describe the purpose of the guideline as 'to provide professionals with a set of practical skills to assess pain as the first step towards its effective management'. They describe how 'assessing pain becomes even more challenging in the presence of severe cognitive impairment, communication difficulties or language and cultural barriers. However, even in the presence of severe cognitive and communication impairment, many individuals may have their pain assessed using appropriate observational scales'.

The key components of an assessment of pain outlined in the National Guidelines are reproduced in Table 4.5.

The Abbey Pain Scale (reproduced in Fig. 4.2) uses some of the behavioural observations highlighted in Table 4.4 earlier in this chapter with a scale indicator of 0–3 to enable pain assessment.

The guideline also incorporates an algorithm for the assessment of pain in older people that has been adapted here (Fig. 4.3) for use when assessing the pain experience of people with learning disability.

The guideline also suggests the use of a 'pain map'. This can be a simple body outline, or can be a more detailed diagram or drawing that a person can use to point at or draw on to indicate a site of pain.

The Abbey Pain Scale does not differentiate between distress and pain and therefore alongside the assessment tool the health care professional must continue to assess the effectiveness of pain-relieving interventions. It also includes examples of different pain scales that could be adapted for your own use. (*Link for Abbey Pain Scale*: www.racgp.org.au/silverbookonline/4–6.asp)

The Abbey Pain Scale
For measurement of pain in people with dementia who cannot verbalise

How to use scale: While observing the resident, score questions 1 to 6.

Name of resident: ....

Name and designation of person completing the scale: ....

Date: ....Time: ....

Latest pain relief given was.. at ....hrs.

Q1. Vocalisation
e.g. whimpering, groaning, crying   Q1 ☐
Absent 0   Mild 1   Moderate 2   Severe 3

Q2. Facial expression
e.g. looking tense, frowning, grimacing, looking frightened   Q2 ☐
Absent 0   Mild 1   Moderate 2   Severe 3

Q3. Change in body language
e.g. fidgeting, rocking, guarding part of body, withdrawn   Q3 ☐
Absent 0   Mild 1   Moderate 2   Severe 3

Q4. Behavioural change
e.g. increased confusion, refusing to eat, alteration in usual patterns   Q4 ☐
Absent 0   Mild 1   Moderate 2   Severe 3

Q5. Physiological change
e.g. temperature, pulse or blood pressure outside normal limits, perspiring, flushing or pallor
Absent 0   Mild 1   Moderate 2   Severe 3   Q5 ☐

Q6. Physical changes
e.g. skin tears, pressure areas, arthritis, contractures, previous injuries   Q6 ☐
Absent 0   Mild 1   Moderate 2   Severe 3

Add scores for Q1 to Q6 and record here   ⇨   Total pain score ☐

Now tick the box that matches
the Total pain score   ⇨

0-2	3-7	8-13	14+
No pain	Mild	Moderate	Severe

Finally, tick the box which matches
the type of pain   ⇨

Chronic	Acute	Acute on chronic

Fig. 4.2   The Abbey Pain scale. Reproduced from Abbey et al. (2007). Funded by the JH & JD Gunn Medical Research Foundation 1998–2002. (This document may be reproduced with this reference retained.)

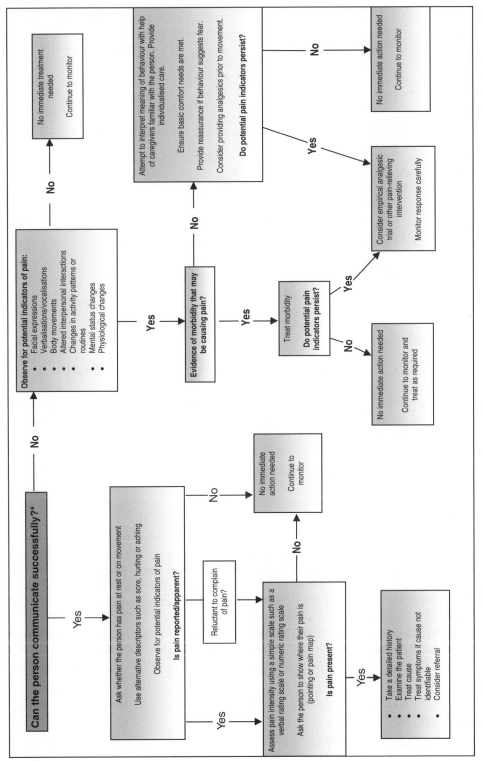

Fig. 4.3 Algorithm for the assessment of pain in people with a learning disability. Reproduced from Royal College of Physicians, British Geriatrics Society and British Pain Society (2007).

Table 4.5 Key components of the assessment of pain

Direct enquiry about the presence of pain
  • including the use of alternative words to describe pain

Observation for signs of pain
  • especially in older people with cognitive/communication impairment

Description of pain to include:
  • sensory dimension
    – the nature of the pain (e.g. sharp, dull, burning etc.)
    – pain location and radiation (by patients pointing to the pain on themselves or by using a pain map)
    – intensity, using a standardised pain assessment scale
  • affective dimension
    – emotional response to pain (e.g. fear, anxiety, depression)
  • impact: disabling effects of pain at the levels of
    – functional activities (e.g. activities of daily living)
    – participation (e.g. work, social activities, relationships)

Measurement of pain
  • using standardised scales in a format that is accessible to the individual

Cause of pain
  • examination and investigation to establish the cause of pain

---

Reproduced from the Royal College of Physicians, British Geriatric Society and Pain Society (2007).

RISK ASSESSMENT

Sometimes an individual's behaviour escalates to a level where they place either themselves or others at risk of harm. This is particularly the case with aggressive and self-injurious behaviour. In these circumstances it is vital that a comprehensive behavioural and risk assessment is completed prior to admission, and expert advice sought from the learning disability service or another relevant health care professional, for example clinical psychologist.

There are three central components to any risk assessment:

1. Significance of the outcome
2. Actions to reduce the risk
3. Recording and review

Specific and detailed risk assessments can be carried out to identify the particular risk behaviours, any potential triggers, and the likelihood of them occurring. The assessment should also include ways of dealing with the behaviour and a planned response of strategies to try. May (2005, p. 43) suggests that 'Being aware of potential triggers and avoiding these as much as possible, as well as watching for indicators that the person is becoming increasingly distressed, can all help in avoiding escalation to a full blown incident'.

Detailed risk management strategies should be developed to minimise, prevent or overcome the risks identified. Good preparation and planning, working together with family/carers who know the person well, will enable even the most difficult behaviours to be successfully coped with.

CONCLUSION

This chapter explores some of the key aspects of understanding behaviour with the aim to help health care professionals understand how the behaviour may have an important function for a person with a learning disability. It highlights how the impact of a hospital admission can affect behaviour and that health care professionals need to develop skills and approaches to enable them to respond to behavioural issues in the hospital setting. The use of behavioural indicators is an important aspect of pain assessment that should be carefully observed.

Summary of Key Learning Points

The key learning points are:

- Around 15% of people with learning disabilities present with some level of challenging behaviour.
- Challenging behaviour is often a way a person communicates how they are feeling.
- To understand the behaviour there needs to be an analysis of the person's circumstances including communication skills, environment, relationships and life events.
- Changes in an individual's behaviour may be due to ill health and/or pain. The first consideration when a person displays a change in behaviour should be to rule out a physical cause.
- Behavioural and psychological approaches are effective in dealing with behavioural issues.
- Positive approaches such as desensitisation or relaxation techniques are effective in managing behavioural issues related to anxiety.
- Physical intervention is sometimes required to manage challenging behaviour. If restraint is considered it must be employed within the legal framework.
- The use of behavioural indicators is important in the assessment of pain in people with a learning disability.
- Risk assessment and careful planning can enable challenging behaviour to be effectively supported in hospital.

Links to KSF Competencies – Chapter 4

	Level descriptors			
Core dimensions	**1**	**2**	**3**	**4**
1 – Communication	Communicate with a limited range of people on day-to-day matters	Communicate with a range of people on a range of matters	Develop and maintain communication with people about difficult matters and/or in difficult situations	Develop and maintain communication with people on complex matters, issues and ideas and/or in complex situations
2 – Personal and people development	Contribute to own personal development	Develop own skills and knowledge and provide information to others to help their development	Develop oneself and contribute to the development of others	Develop oneself and others in areas of practice
3 – Health safety and security	Assist in maintaining own and others' health, safety and security	Monitor and maintain health, safety and security of self and others	Promote, monitor and maintain best practice in health, safety and security	Maintain and develop an environment and culture that improves health, safety and security

4 – Service improvement	Make changes in own practice and offer suggestions for improving services	Contribute to the improvement of services	Appraise, interpret and apply suggestions, recommendations and directives to improve services	Work in partnership with others to develop, take forward and evaluate direction, policies and strategies
5 – Quality	Maintain the quality of own work	Maintain quality in own work and encourage others to do so	Contribute to improving quality	Develop a culture that improves quality
6 – Equality and diversity	Act in ways that support equality and value diversity	Support equality and value diversity	Promote equality and value diversity	Develop a culture that promotes equality and values diversity

Health and well-being	Level descriptors			
	1	2	3	4
HWB1 – Promotion of health and well-being and prevention of adverse effects on health and well-being	Contribute to promoting health and well-being and preventing adverse effects on health and well-being	Plan, develop and implement approaches to promote health and well-being and prevent adverse effects on health and well-being	Plan, develop and implement programmes to promote health and well-being and prevent adverse effects on health and well-being	Promote health and well-being and prevent adverse effects on health and well-being through contributing to the development, implementation and evaluation of related policies
HWB2 – Assessment and care planning to meet health and well-being needs	Assist in the assessment of people's health and well-being needs	Contribute to assessing health and well-being needs and planning how to meet those needs	Assess health and well-being needs and develop, monitor and review care plans to meet specific needs	Assess complex health and well-being needs and develop, monitor and review care plans to meet those needs
HWB3 – Protection of health and well-being	Recognise and report situations where there might be a need for protection	Contribute to protecting people at risk	Implement aspects of a protection plan and review its effectiveness	Develop and lead on the implementation of an overall protection plan
HWB4 – Enablement to address health and well-being needs	Help people meet daily health and well-being needs	Enable people to meet ongoing health and well-being needs	Enable people to address specific needs in relation to health and well-being	Empower people to realise and maintain their potential in relation to health and well-being

HWB5 – Provision of care to meet health and well-being needs	Undertake care activities to meet individuals' health and well-being needs	Undertake care activities to meet the health and well-being needs of individuals with a greater degree of dependency	Plan, deliver and evaluate care to meet people's health and well-being needs	Plan, deliver and evaluate care to address people's complex health and well-being needs
HWB6 – Assessment and treatment planning	Undertake tasks related to the assessment of physiological and psychological functioning	Contribute to the assessment of physiological and psychological functioning	Assess physiological and psychological functioning and develop, monitor and review related treatment plans	Assess physiological and psychological functioning when there are complex and/or undifferentiated abnormalities, diseases and disorders and develop, monitor and review related treatment plans
HWB7 – Interventions and treatments	Assist in providing interventions and/or treatments	Contribute to planning, delivering and monitoring interventions and/or treatments	Plan, deliver and evaluate interventions and/or treatments	Plan, deliver and evaluate interventions and/or treatments when there are complex issues and/or serious illness

Department of Health (2005). Reproduced under the terms of the Click-Use Licence.

REFERENCES

Abbey J, De Bellis A, Piller N et al. (2007) Abbey pain scale. In: *The Royal Australian College of General Practitioners – 'Silver Book' National Taskforce. Medical Care of Older Persons in Residential Aged Care Facilities.*

Astor R (2001) Detecting pain in people with profound learning disabilities. *Nursing Standard*, 97(40), 38.

Blundell R and Allen D (1987) *Facing the Challenge: An Ordinary Life for People with Learning Difficulties and Challenging Behaviour*. Kings Fund Paper No. 74. Kings Fund, London.

British Institute of Learning Disabilities (2002) *Ethical Approaches to Physical Interventions*. BILD, Kidderminster.

British Institute of Learning Disabilities (BILD) (2008) *Physical Interventions: A Policy Framework*, second edition. BILD, Kidderminster.

Brittle R (2004) Managing the needs of people who have a learning disability. *Nursing Times*, 100(10), 28–29.

Clements J and Zarkowska E (2000) *Behavioural Concerns and Autistic Spectrum Disorders: Explanations and Strategies for Change*. Jessica Kingsley Publishers, London.

Davis D and Evans L (2001) Assessing pain in people with profound learning disabilities. *British Journal of Nursing*, 10(8), 513–516.

Department of Health (1983) *Mental Health Act*. HMSO, London.

Department of Health (2004) *The NHS Knowledge and Skills Framework (NHS KSF) and the Development Review Process. Appendix 1: Overview of the NHS KSF*. HMSO, London.

Department of Health (2005) *Mental Capacity Act*. HMSO, London.

Disability Rights Commission (DRC) (2006) *Equal Treatment: Closing the Gap*. DRC, London.

Emerson E, Cummings R, Barrett S, Hughes H and McCod S (1998) Challenging behaviour and community services: who are the people who challenge services? *Mental Handicap*, 16, 11–19.

Foley P and McClutcheon H (2004) Detecting pain in people with an intellectual disability. *Accident and Emergency Nursing*, 12(4), 196–200.

Gates B, Gear J and Wray J (2000) *Behavioural Distress, Concepts and Strategies*. Bailliere Tindall, London.

Gordon SM, Dionne RA and Snyder DD (1998) Dental fear and anxiety as a barrier to accessing health care among patients with special health care needs. *Special Care Dentist*, 18, 288–292.

Grant G, Goward P, Richardson M and Ramcharan P (2005) *Learning Disability: A life Cycle Approach to Valuing People*. Open University Press, Maidenhead, England.

Hannon L (2003) Pre-admission assessment in secondary healthcare services for people with learning disabilities. Unpublished MSc Dissertation. University of Central Lancashire.

Hewitt D (ed.) (2001) *Challenging Behaviour: Principles and Practices*. David Fulton Publishing, London.

Kelly A (2000) *Working with Adults with a learning Disability*. Wimslow Press, Oxon.

Lebus JS, Keefe FJ and Jensen MP (2003) Self-reports of pain intensity and direct observations of pain behaviour: when are they correlated? *Pain*, 102(1–2), 109–124.

Lovett H (1996) *Learning to Listen: Positive Approaches and People with Difficult Behaviour*. Jessica Kingsley Publishing, London.

Lyon C and Pimor A (2004) *Physical Interventions and the Law. Legal Issues from the Use of Physical Interventions in Supporting Children, Young People and Adults with Learning Disabilities and Severe Challenging Behaviour*. BILD, Kidderminster.

May F (2005) *Understanding Behaviour*. National Autistic Society, London.

Mencap (2007) *Death by Indifference*. Mencap, London.

Michaels J (2008) *Healthcare for All. Report of the Independent Inquiry into Access to Healthcare for People with Learning Disabilities*. HMSO, London.

Moss S, Emerson E, Kiernan C, Turner S, Hatton C and Alborz A (2000) Psychiatric symptoms in adults with learning disability and challenging behaviour. *British Journal of Psychiatry*, 177, 452–456.

Murphy G, Kelly-Pike A and McGill P (2002) Psychiatric symptoms in adults with learning disability and challenging behaviour. *British Journal of Psychiatry*, 177, 452–456.

Northumberland Tyne & Wear NHS Trust and St. Oswald's Hospice (2008) *Disability Distress Assessment Tool* (DisDAT), Vol. 19.

Parliamentary and Health Service Ombudsman (2009) *Six Lives: The Provision of Public Services to People with Learning Disabilities*. The Stationery Office, London.

Prangell SJ and Green K (2008) A cognitive behavioural intervention for dental anxiety for people with learning disabilities: a case study. *British Journal of Learning Disabilities*, 36, 242–248.

Regnard C, Reynolds J, Watson B, Matthews D, Gibson L and Clarke C (2007) Understanding distress in people with severe communication difficulties: developing and assessing the disability distress assessment tool (DisDAT). *Journal of Intellectual Disability Research*, 51(4), 277–292.

Royal College of Nursing Institute (1999) *Clinical Practice Guidelines: The Recognition and Assessment of Acute Pain in Children – Recommendations*. Royal College of Nursing, London.

Royal College of Physicians (RCP), British Geriatrics Society and British Pain Society (2007) *The Assessment of Pain in Older People: National Guidelines*. Concise guidance to good practice series (number 8). RCP, London.

University College, London/Institute of Child Health and the Royal College of Nursing (RCN) Institute (2003) *Paediatric Pain Profile*. RCN, London.

Wood S (2008) Pain assessment; assessment and diagnosis for successful pain management. *Nursing Times*, September 2008. Available at www.nursingtimes.net/nursing=practice-clinical-research/assessment-of-pain/1861174. Article last accessed July 2009.

5 Consent

INTRODUCTION

The area of consent often presents complex and difficult issues for health care professionals working with people with a learning disability. Everyone has a fundamental legal and ethical right to decide what happens to their own body, and a person with a learning disability has exactly the same rights as anyone else. In law, people aged 16 or more are assumed to have the ability to make decisions about their own health care and their consent to treatment is required before you can proceed.

Valid consent is central to the health care process as it is the agreement between the patient and the health professional to provide care. This consent covers every aspect of health, ranging from providing personal care to undertaking major surgery. Health care professionals are often unsure about how to obtain this consent from a person with a learning disability, and how much they actually understand about the health care process.

It should be clearly understood that before any health care is initiated, consent must be obtained from the patient. Obtaining consent should not be seen as just a one-off event, as patients should be informed throughout their assessment and treatment to ensure that they fully understand the care that they are receiving, and are able to withdraw their consent at any time if they wish to do so.

This chapter explores the consent process from the perspective of a patient who has learning disabilities. For those of you who have already experienced the difficulties of supporting a patient who is refusing treatment, or if you have felt concern that the intervention or treatment has not been fully explained, we hope that the following information will help you.

WHAT DO WE MEAN BY CONSENT?

Consent is a patient's agreement for the health care professional to provide them with health care. The patient may do this verbally, or in writing, or the consent may be indicated non-verbally by passive acceptance or compliance with the health care procedure (e.g. holding out an arm for a blood test). The health care professional must always be satisfied that the patient is consenting before proceeding with providing health care.

General Hospital Care for People with Learning Disabilities, *First Edition* by Lynn Hannon and Julie Clift
© 2011 Blackwell Publishing Ltd

For this consent to be valid the patient must:

- Be competent to make that decision
- Have received sufficient information to make the decision
- Not be acting under duress

The Royal College of Nursing (RCN 2006, p. 8) explains that 'In the past it was assumed that having learning disabilities meant people lacked the capacity to make decisions. However, it is now recognised that people with learning disabilities have as much right to make decisions for themselves as anyone else'. They outline that the UK has two separate laws on capacity to consent:

- The Mental Capacity Act 2005 in England and Wales (Department for Constitutional Affairs 2005)
- Adults with Incapacity Act 2000 in Scotland (Scottish Executive 2000)

They also explain that 'although the Acts and case law differ in terminology and procedures they are based on similar principles and have similar expectations of health care staff. The underlying principles in both Acts are that no adult can make a decision on behalf of another adult, and it must be assumed that a person has the capacity to make a decision unless proved otherwise. Adults, with or without learning disabilities can refuse examination or treatment, even if it is detrimental to their health, as long as they have the capacity to do so'.

The RCN continues to state that 'It is the responsibility of the lead professional (i.e. the person who is likely to undertake the examination or instigate the treatment) who is responsible for assessing whether a person has the capacity to make a decision about examination or treatment'.

Reflective Learning Point:

What are the important issues you would consider about obtaining consent if you were asked to provide treatment to a person with a learning disability?

Every registered health care professional is required to abide by a professional code of conduct that governs the standards of their professional practice and also offers guidance about consent. As it is not possible to cover every code within this book we have chosen to use the Nursing and Midwifery code of conduct as an example, though each health care professional will need to make reference to their own specific code in practice.

In 2008 issued *The Code: Standards of Conduct, Performance and Ethics for Nurses and Midwives*. The NMC code of conduct governs nursing practice and acts a practical and ethical guide to practice. The document covers legal, ethical and professional guidance in areas of consent, confidentiality and collaborative working.

The NMC code makes it clear that in caring for patients and clients the registered nurse, midwife or specialist community public health nurse must:

- Treat people as individuals
- Respect people's confidentiality

- Collaborate with those in your care
- Ensure you gain consent
- Maintain clear professional boundaries
- Share information with your colleagues
- Work effectively as part of a team
- Delegate effectively
- Manage risk
- Use the best available evidence
- Keep your skills and knowledge up to date
- Keep clear and accurate records
- Act with integrity
- Deal with problems
- Be impartial
- Uphold the reputation of your profession

With particular reference to consent the NMC code advises:

- You must ensure that you gain consent before you begin any treatment or care.
- You must respect and support people's rights to accept or decline treatment and care.
- You must uphold people's rights to be fully involved in decisions about their care.
- You must be aware of the legislation regarding mental capacity, ensuring that people who lack capacity remain at the centre of decision making and are fully safeguarded.
- You must be able to demonstrate that you have acted in someone's best interests if you have provided care in an emergency.

The issue of consent can present many practical and ethical dilemmas for health care professionals, and careful consideration needs to be given when obtaining informed consent from any patient. Even more consideration is needed when obtaining consent from a person with a learning disability. (You will find more information in Chapter 1 about how to establish if your patient has a learning disability.)

ETHICAL DECISION MAKING

Ethical dilemmas occur frequently when supporting people with learning disabilities especially when it is not clear what the right thing to do is. Ethical dilemmas are most problematic when a number of different people have a view on what should be the preferred course of action. In some situations there may be the discussion as to whether the intervention is ethical or morally right. This is especially apparent in decision making about decisions to withhold treatment, such as resuscitation, and quality of life.

Take the following scenario for example: One area that often raises ethical dilemmas is the management of menstruation and contraception for women who have profound learning disabilities. The need for the use of medication, surgical sterilisation, and on occasions, hysterectomy to relieve the symptoms of menstruation or to prevent the risk of pregnancy occasionally rises. These situations often raise issues around the rights of the individual. The historical practice of routinely sterilising people with learning disabilities without their consent could not happen within the current legal framework, and raises many ethical issues even nowadays.

It is a good practice to involve an appropriately trained professional with learning disability experience, possibly a Consultant Psychiatrist, in the multi-disciplinary decision making in these cases, especially where there are concerns raised by any member of that team.

Where it is clear that the treatment option is the least invasive and is the most therapeutic response, with all parties involved in the decision making are happy to proceed, then no further legal action would be required. However, if there is any disagreement then the case would need to be referred to the court for them to make the decision.

Griffith and Tengnah (2008, p. 21) state that 'Morals are influenced not only by the law but by our culture, religion and experience'. Morals are based on your values and beliefs and this will influence your decision making when caring for a person. This statement can be applied to the care of any individual, but your values and beliefs are likely to raise even more issues to consider when supporting a person with a learning disability.

When supporting people with learning disabilities making decisions about their health care there may be occasions where you find that some clinical decisions are not morally acceptable to you. This is particularly relevant when decisions are made on the basis of quality-of-life issues.

Consent Case Study 1 – Susan

Susan has been admitted to hospital with aspiration pneumonia. She has profound learning disabilities and limited mobility so she uses a wheel chair. She has been assessed as not for resuscitation by her doctor and the high dependency care team with the agreement of her next of kin (who does not live with Susan and only has contact four times a year). You have spoken with her carers who are concerned that this decision is based on her quality of life due to her having a learning disability.

The key issues here are about the severity of her pneumonia and how this would normally be treated, and the consideration of who is best placed to inform the decision maker about Susan's quality of life. The ethical dilemma is around considering the impact of treatment on a person who has profound and physical disabilities, who is in a wheelchair and with high levels of care needs. The judgement is about the ongoing quality of life for the person, balanced with clinical need.

The decision maker should speak with those people most concerned with Susan's care, that is, her carers, although the next of kin also needs to be involved in this process. Consideration should be given to what the impact of receiving or not receiving the treatment would have on her ongoing quality of life. This should be judged on what is acceptable for her, based on the opinion of all parties, and then a decision is made on a clinical basis, taking this opinion into account.

(Quality of life issues are discussed further later in this chapter, and ethical issues are explored in Chapter 6.)

The four principles framework

Beauchamp and Childress (1989) provide a 'four principles' approach for exploring moral reasoning in health care that can be expanded to apply to various ethical conflicts and dilemmas.

The four principles are:

- *Principle 1 – Respect for autonomy*: Enabling individuals to make informed choices and respecting the person's decision-making capacity.

- *Principle 2 – Beneficence*: Balancing the risks and benefits of treatment and care in a way that is of benefit for the person.
- *Principle 3 – Non-malfeasance*: Avoiding harm – any harm caused as a result of the treatment or care must not be disproportionate to the benefits of the treatment or care.
- *Principle 4 – Justice*: Patients in similar situations must be treated in the same way.

The following case study illustrates the use of these four principles as a guide to enable informed decision making when working with people with a learning disability.

Consent Case Study 2 – Joanne

Joanne is 56 years old and has a learning disability. Joanne has endometriosis. The endometriosis is causing a blockage in her ureter and this is having an effect on her renal function. If left untreated this condition may result in renal failure. Joanne would need an operation to reduce the impact of the endometriosis on her ureter. The surgeon assesses that Joanne does not have the capacity to make this decision.

Joanne is needle phobic and her carer is concerned that Joanne will refuse treatment based on her fear of needles. If Joanne does not have the surgery she may develop renal failure and require dialysis which would involve the regular use of needles and be very difficult to carry out given her fear of needles. Joanne tells her carer that she does not want to go into hospital and have an operation because of the needles.

Respect for autonomy

The principle of respect for autonomy entails taking into account and giving consideration to Joanne's views on her treatment. Joanne may not be fully autonomous as she does not have the capacity to make this decision, but this does not mean that ethically her views should not be considered and respected as far as possible. She has expressed that she does not want to go into hospital because of the needles. Although this is Joanne's decision not to go into hospital we need to establish if she has been given enough information, in a manner that she can comprehend, to be able to make an informed choice. This may include considering other aspects of her care that she can understand, for example: Would she prefer to walk to theatre or go on a trolley? What would she like to take to hospital with her?

Beneficence

In deciding how to ensure that we are providing treatment and care in a way that benefits Joanne we should consider both the long-term and short-term effects of overriding Joanne's views. Joanne will be frightened when she has to have a needle inserted in her arm. Using restraint to insert a needle may in the short term lead her to distrust health care professionals in the future. However, in the long term there will be a benefit to Joanne having her autonomy overridden on this occasion as without this surgery it is likely that she will suffer serious and long-term health problems that would require dialysis. Therefore the decision to carry on with treatment in her best interest is, on balance, of greater importance than acting to promote Joanne's autonomy not to have treatment.

Non-malfeasance

This requires the health care professional to do no harm to the patient. In this situation, Joanne may be harmed by forcibly restraining her in order to insert the needle prior to anaesthetic. If she is not treated now she may require dialysis a number of times per week which will require her to have a needle inserted. This decision relies on assumptions: How successful is the operation likely to be? How likely will Joanne comply with dialysis? Which option is likely to result in the least harm to Joanne?

Justice
How would this situation be managed with another patient in a similar situation? Would the decision be the same?

It may also be necessary to consider the economic cost of the surgical option over lifelong dialysis.

The issues highlighted in this case study may be familiar to many health care professionals. You may have also taken part in ethical discussions where you did or did not agree with the final decision.

Reflective Learning Point:

- How would you approach this situation in your own area of work with consideration of each of these four principles?
- What would help you to feel that you had made the right decision?

THE LAW ON CONSENT AND CAPACITY TO CONSENT (IN ENGLAND AND WALES)

The main legislation that covers consent and capacity to consent are:

- Mental Capacity Act 2005 (Department for Constitutional Affairs 2005)
- Human Rights Act 1998 (Department of Health 1998)
- Disability Discrimination Act 1995 (Department of Health 2005)

The Mental Capacity Act 2005

The Mental Capacity Act (MCA) 2005 provides 'a framework for people who lack capacity to make decisions for themselves, or who have capacity and want to make preparations for a time when they may lack capacity in the future. It sets out who can take decisions, in which situations, and how they should go about this'.

The Act applies to people aged 16 and more in England and Wales. The NMC newsletter in February 2009 included a briefing paper on the Act which explained that the Act tells people:

- What to do to help someone make their own decisions about something
- How to work out if someone can make their own decisions about something
- What to do if someone cannot make decisions about something

In the MCA 2005, a person's capacity (or lack of capacity) refers specifically to their capacity to make a particular decision at the time it needs to be made. A finding of 'lack of capacity' cannot be made merely on the basis of a person's age or appearance, or from assumptions based on the person's condition or any aspect of his or her behaviour.

The fact that a patient has a learning disability does *not* alter the need to obtain informed consent. This may cause concerns when the health care professional is unclear whether the person with the learning disability has the capacity to understand the implications of the procedure they are being asked to consent to.

It should not be assumed that because the person has a learning disability that they cannot give consent. It is, therefore, vital for health care professionals to recognise that *in most cases* consent should be sought from the patient themselves.

Who does the MCA 2005 apply to?

The legal framework of the MCA, supported by the code of practice (Department for Constitutional Affairs 2007), provides guidance for health care professionals when working with or caring for adults who may lack capacity to make decisions for themselves. The code has 'statutory force' which means that certain categories of people are legally required to 'have regard to' the guidance in it when making decisions for people who lack the capacity to be able to make the decision for themselves.

- People working in a professional capacity with a person who lacks capacity
- People who are paid to care or support a person who lacks capacity
- Anyone who is a deputy or appointed by the Court of Protection
- An attorney under a lasting power of attorney (LPA)
- Anyone acting as an independent mental capacity advocate (IMCA)
- Anyone carrying out research involving people who lack capacity

These categories cover a variety of health care staff and anyone else who may be involved in the care of people who lack capacity.

The MCA 2005 does not impose a legal duty on anyone to comply with the code, but should be viewed as best practice guidance. However, if a health care professional does not apply the principles and guidance outlined in the code, then they will be expected to be able to give good justification as to why they have chosen not to follow the code of practice.

Making decisions for another person

Power of attorney

In the UK, it is *not legal* for a parent or carer to give consent on behalf of an adult with a learning disability; however, the MCA 2005 does allow for third parties to make decisions on behalf of a person who lacks decision-making capacity. The power can be given to a designated decision maker to have the right to make decisions to consent or refuse medical treatment.

The only people who have this right – other than those who normally are involved in the persons care – are:

- Attorneys under an LPA
- Court-appointed deputies

Lasting power of attorney

The power to give consent for health treatment on behalf of a person who lacks capacity to make decisions can be given through a *personal welfare lasting power of attorney*. The MCA code (p. 115) describes a power of attorney as 'a legal document that means one person gives another person authority to make a decision on their behalf'.

Under the LPA an individual (the donor) can appoint another person to act on their behalf in relation to certain decisions regarding their financial, health and welfare matters.

There are two types of LPA:

1. Personal welfare (including health care and consent to treatment)
2. Property and affairs (including financial matters)

Attorneys acting under an LPA have a duty to:

- Follow the MCA statutory principles (see section on MCA)
- Make decisions in the donor's best interests
- Have regard to the guidance in the MCA code of practice
- Only make decisions the LPA gives them authority to make

Even where the LPA includes health care decisions the attorney does not have the right to consent or refuse treatment where:

- The donor has capacity to make the decision
- The donor has made an advance decision to refuse treatment
- A decision relates to life-sustaining treatment
- The donor is detained under the Mental Health Act 1983 (Department of Health 1999)

LPAs replace the enduring power of attorney (EPA) introduced in the Enduring Powers of Attorney Act (1985). EPAs only cover property and affairs and did not include personal welfare issues. Whilst it is not possible now to make new EPAs, existing (valid) EPAs can still be used. Some people (if they still have capacity) may choose to cancel the EPA and make a new LPA.

If you are working with a patient where a designated decision maker with authority is in place, they must give their consent before care or treatment can be given.

(For further information about LPA, see MCA, Sections 9–14; MCA (2007) code of practice, Chapter 7)

The Court of Protection and court-appointed deputies

It is expected that the Court of Protection will only be involved where particularly difficult disputes are involved. For example, to determine if a proposed action is lawful, or the decision is in the person's best interest, and the meaning or effect of an LPA in disputed cases.

The Court of Protection has powers to:

- Decide whether a person has capacity to make a decision themselves
- Make declarations, decisions or orders affecting people who lack capacity
- Appoint deputies to make decisions for people lacking capacity
- Decide whether an LPA or an EPA is valid
- Remove deputies or attorneys who fail to carry out their duties

MCA code (2007, p. 137)

Cases involving the following serious health care and treatment decisions should always be brought before the court:

- The proposed withholding or withdrawal of artificial nutrition and hydration from patients in a permanent vegetative state
- Organ or bone marrow donation by a person who lacks consent
- The proposed non-therapeutic sterilisation of a person who lacks capacity
- All other cases where there is a doubt or dispute about 'best interests'

Court-appointed deputies

Court-appointed deputies are appointed by the Court of Protection to make ongoing decisions for the person who lacks capacity. The MCA code (2007, p. 148) states that 'Deputies for personal welfare (including health care) decisions will only be required in the most difficult cases where:

- Important and necessary actions cannot be carried out without the court's authority, or
- There is no other way of settling a best interests matter'

A deputy can be a family member, someone who knows the person well, or any other person the court thinks suitable, and must always act with regard to the MCA code of practice. In some cases, the court will appoint a deputy who is completely independent, and on occasions, a professional deputy, for example where someone's affairs or care needs are particularly complicated. Paid care workers should not generally be appointed as deputies and conflict of interest should also be considered by the court.

(For further information about the Court of Protection and Court-appointed deputies, see (MCA (2007) part 2; code of practice, Chapter 8.)

Human Rights Act 1998

The Human Rights Act (HRA) is a law that largely incorporates the substantive rights set out in the European Convention of Human Rights into UK law. There are 17 Articles within the European convention covering a range of rights and freedoms that every individual is entitled to. In the provision of health care and decisions around capacity to consent, the main article for consideration within the HRA is Article 5 – the right to liberty and security.

Article 5 outlines a right to 'freedom of movement' and states that 'everyone has a right to liberty and security of person'. In health care, this could mean the potential for depriving a person of their liberty by the use of restraint in order to impose treatment.

The European Court of Human Rights and UK courts have determined a number of factors that can be relevant when making decisions about the use of restraint or deprivation of liberty in the process of the delivery of care and treatment of people who lack capacity to consent.

These factors are as follows:

- If restraint is used, including sedation, to admit a person to an institution where that person is resisting admission.
- Staff exercise complete and effective control over the care and movement of a person for a significant period.
- Staff exercise control over assessments, treatment, contacts and residence.
- A decision has been taken by the institution that the person will not be released into the care of others, or permitted to live elsewhere, unless the staff in the institution consider it appropriate.
- A request by carers for a person to be discharged to their care is refused.
- The person is unable to maintain social contacts because of restrictions placed on their access to other people.
- The person loses autonomy because they are under continuous supervision and control.

Ministry of Justice (2008, p. 17) (*See also section on restraint and physical intervention in Chapter 4.*)

Disability Discrimination Act 1995 and 2005

People with disabilities now have rights under the Disability Discrimination Act (DDA) to address the discrimination they experience in areas such as health and social care, education and employment.

We do not always know who is disabled. Many people associate disability with wheelchair use, yet less than 5% of disabled people use a wheelchair. Anyone who meets the following definition from the DDA is considered to be disabled:

> Someone with a *physical* or *mental impairment* which has a *substantial* and *long-term* adverse effect on their ability to carry out normal *day-to-day activities*.

This includes *physical impairments* to senses such as sight and hearing, and *mental impairments* such as learning disabilities and mental illness. Conditions covered may include things like severe depression, diabetes, dyslexia, cardiovascular diseases, epilepsy and arthritis.

Substantial includes:

- Inability to see moving traffic clearly enough to cross a road in safety
- Inability to turn taps or knobs
- Inability to remember and relay a simple message correctly

Long-term means that the effects have lasted, or are expected to last 12 months or more.

Day-to-day activities include mobility, manual dexterity, physical coordination, continence, ability to lift, speech, hearing, eyesight, memory and recognising physical danger.

It is important for health care professionals to be able to identify what constitutes discrimination and have an awareness of the requirements within the Act to support disabled people in their care. All service providers have a duty under the DDA to ensure that they do not discriminate against people with disabilities by:

- Refusing to provide a service, or deliberately not providing, any service they provide to the general public
- The standard of the service or the manner in which the service is provided
- The terms on which the service is provided

Services are also required to make *reasonable adjustments* to services, premises, employment conditions or courses of education to enable the disabled person to access the service equitably.

Reasonable adjustments to service are an important component when providing any service to people with a learning disability as their needs may be significantly different from the mainstream population. This can sometimes include simple things for example, giving someone a first appointment in a clinic to avoid busy waiting areas and the patient having to wait due to clinic delays, or using pictures to illustrate a health procedure. (*Further advice on accessible information can be found in Chapter 3.*)

DEFINING CAPACITY

Capacity can be defined as 'The ability to make decisions about a particular matter at the time the decision needs to be made' MCA 2005 code of practice (2007). This reflects the fact that 'people may lack capacity to make some decisions for themselves, but will have capacity to make other decisions'.

A person may be able to make a decision at a later date if their capacity changes. The Act also reflects the fact that 'while some people may always lack capacity to make some kind of decisions – for example, due to a condition or severe learning disability that has affected them from birth – others may learn new skills that enable them to gain capacity and make decisions for themselves'.

People with a learning disability might have difficulty in understanding information, depending on how it is presented to them, and it is the health care professionals' responsibility to take all necessary steps to support the person in making the decision. The MCA code (2007, p. 29) states that 'Before deciding that someone lacks capacity to make a particular decision, it is important to take all practical and appropriate steps to enable them to make that decision themselves'. Person-centred planning is suggested as a way of providing help with decision making for people with learning disabilities. (*See Chapter 1 for further information about this.*)

All Capacity Assessments are 'decision specific'.

This means that the assessment of capacity must be based only on the person's ability to make a specific decision at the time it needs to be made. The decision regarding capacity is not to be based on a global generalisation of understanding. For example, the patient may be able to choose to have either tea or coffee, or make the decision of what they would like to watch on the television, probably based on previous experience, but they would not be able to make a complex decision about serious medical treatment.

The RCN (2006, p. 9) highlights that 'Capacity can change over time. If a person was previously unable to make a decision it should not be assumed that they still cannot. Some people may be able to make some decisions, but have difficulty with others, so it is important that each decision is treated independently'.

The MCA code (2007) provides the following quick summary of points which may be helpful to consider in making your assessment and decision:

- Providing relevant information:
  - Does the person have all the relevant information they need to make a particular decision?
  - If they have a choice, have they been given information on all the alternatives?
- Communicating in an appropriate way:
  - Could information be explained or presented in a way that is easier for the person to understand (e.g. using simple language or visual aids)
  - Have different methods of communication been explored if required, including non-verbal communication?
  - Could anyone else help with communication (e.g. a family member, support worker, interpreter, speech and language therapist or advocate)?
- Making the person feel at ease:
  - Are there particular times of day when the person's understanding is better?
  - Are there particular locations where they may feel more at ease?
  - Could the decision be put off to see whether the person can make the decision at a later time when circumstances are right for them?
- Supporting the person:
  - Can anyone else help or support the person to make choices or express a view?

When considering if a person has the capacity to give consent, health care professionals should ensure that they are familiar with the (2007) MCA 2005 code of practice, and be able to provide evidence that if they make decisions to act on behalf of a patient who lacks capacity, that they have acted in their best interests. If a person is assessed as lacking capacity, health care professionals can still provide treatment as long as they can demonstrate it is in their best interests. This may also involve consultation with family and carers.

Section 1 of the MCA 2005 sets out *five statutory principles*, which are described in the code of practice as 'the values that underpin the legal requirements of the act'. The five statutory principles are as follows:

1. A person must be assumed to have capacity unless it is established that they lack capacity.
2. A person is not to be treated as unable to make a decision unless all practicable steps to help them to do so have been taken without success.
3. A person is not to be treated as unable to make a decision merely because they make an unwise decision.
4. An act done, or decision made, under this act for or on behalf of a person who lacks capacity must be done, or made, in their best interest.

5. Before the act is done, or the decision is made, regard must be had to whether the purpose for which it is needed can be as effectively achieved in a way that is less restrictive of the person's rights and freedom of action.

These are the key principles on which all health care professionals must base their actions before providing any health care intervention.

When is an assessment of capacity required?

The fact that a person has a learning disability does not necessarily mean that they do not have the capacity to give consent and every effort should be made to enable an informed decision to be made by the individual. You should always start from an assumption that a person has capacity and only consider further assessment if any doubts then arise.

Doubts about a person's capacity to make a decision can occur because of:

- *The person's behaviour*: For example, the person is unable to give you the information you require to assess their needs, or appears not to understand what you are saying.
- *Their circumstances*: For example, a person who attends with a parent or carer who relies on these people to explain what is happening.
- *Concerns raised by someone else*: The family/carer suggests that the person is unable to understand what is happening.

Any doubts must be thoroughly investigated before you proceed to provide care. (*See also information in Chapter 1 on how to tell if your patient has a learning disability.*)

The RCN (2006) highlights that 'The assessment determines whether the person understands and retains the information about the decision; that they are able to weigh and balance the information to make a choice; and they are able to communicate that choice through whatever means of communication the person uses (verbal, sign language, written)'.

Reflective Learning Point:

- What would help you to decide that a person had capacity to make decisions about health care?
- How would you approach this decision with a person with a learning disability?

Who assesses mental capacity?

Generally mental capacity is assessed, when necessary, as part of the usual health needs assessment process. The person who is required to assess an individual's capacity will be the person who intends to take some action in connection with the person's care, or who is contemplating making a decision on the person's behalf.

It will therefore depend on the particular circumstances, but for most day-to-day actions, or decisions, it is expected that the carer most directly involved with the person at the time will assess his or her capacity to make the decision in question. Alternatively a professional such as a doctor, nurse or social worker may be involved where decisions about care arrangements, accommodation or treatment have to be made. In most circumstances, it is sufficient for the person assessing capacity to hold a reasonable belief that the person lacks capacity to make a decision.

The more significant the decision, the more formal the assessment of capacity may need to be. For example, in matters of serious medical treatment a professional, such as a psychiatrist or psychologist, may be asked for an opinion to assist with the assessment. A professional opinion may help to justify a finding about capacity, but the decision as to whether someone has or lacks capacity must be taken by the potential decision-maker or person taking the action, and not the professional who is merely there to give advice.

If you are required to make a judgement about someone's capacity to accept or decline treatment, you need to decide whether the person understands the information you are giving them, and is able to use that information to make that particular decision.

You should use the following guidance to assist this process.

Assessment of capacity

A four-stage assessment process is outlined by Griffith and Tengnah (2008):

1. *The trigger phase*: You must assume that a patient 16 years or older has capacity to consent to care or treatment unless a concern triggers a doubt about the person's decision-making capacity.
2. *The practical support phase*: You cannot say a person lacks decision-making capacity unless you have taken practical steps to help them make a decision.
3. *The diagnostic threshold*: Are you able to discern an impairment or disturbance to the functioning of the person's mind or brain? It does not matter if this is permanent or temporary. If you cannot determine such an impairment or disturbance, no further action can be taken under the MCA 2005.
4. *The assessment phase*: How far does the impairment or disturbance to the person's mind or brain affect their ability to make a decision? Where a person cannot
   - Understand treatment information; or
   - Retain treatment information; or
   - Use or weigh treatment information when making a decision; or
   - Communicate their decision in some way, then you can reasonably conclude that they lack capacity for that particular decision.

Where you have any doubts about a person's capacity, best practice advice within the MCA 2005 and its principles for assessment, is to proceed to carry out the following test.

The two-stage test

Stage 1: Is there an impairment of, or disturbance in, the functioning of the persons mind or brain?

Stage 2: If so is the impairment or disturbance sufficient that the person lacks the capacity to make *that particular decision*?

It is important to highlight the stage 2 test because the MCA (2005) states that 'the person suggesting that the patient lacks capacity has proof that "on the balance of probability" the patient lacks capacity at that time to make that particular decision'. Whilst a person may be considered to lack capacity to make some decisions the same cannot be automatically applied to other decisions they have to make.

Involving other professionals

Any of the following factors might indicate the need for other professional involvement in assessing mental capacity:

- The decision that needs to be made is complicated or has serious consequences
- An assessor concludes a person lacks capacity, and the person challenges the finding
- Family members, carers and/or professionals disagree about a person's capacity
- The person being assessed is expressing different views to different people, perhaps in an effort to please everyone or to tell them what they want to hear
- Somebody might challenge the person's capacity to make the decision, either at the time the decision is made or in the future – for example a person's will might be challenged after their death
- Somebody has been accused of abusing a vulnerable adult who may lack capacity to make decisions that protect them
- A person is repeatedly making decisions that put him or her at risk or could result in preventable suffering or damage.

Other professionals who may be able to help with the assessment process include psychologist, psychiatrist, learning disability nurse, social worker, IMCA, and any other health care professional with knowledge of the treatment under discussion.

OBTAINING CONSENT

At the beginning of this chapter we explained that for consent to be valid the patient must:

- Be competent to make that decision
- Have received sufficient information to make the decision
- Not be acting under duress

It is important to note that an adult who is considered to have decision-making capacity can refuse treatment, even if they know that not receiving the treatment may lead to their death.

The individual's competency to give consent is discussed earlier in this chapter, and the focus of responsibility is on the health care professional involved to provide the necessary information that the individual needs to give their consent, in a format that they can understand. (*This issue is addressed further in Chapter 3.*)

It is also the responsibility of the health care professional to ensure that the individual makes the decision freely, and not by anyone putting any pressure on them to make a certain choice. This pressure may be brought by health care professionals, or by family or carers who may believe they know what the individual should decide.

When attempting to obtain informed consent the health care professional involved should consider carefully the patient's level of understanding and comprehension – it may be appropriate to involve contacting people who have a detailed knowledge of the patient. The use of language and presentation of information should be appropriate to the patient and may require adaptation to complement the verbal and written information.

Expressed consent

Expressed consent can be obtained in two ways – verbal or written:

- *Verbal*: The patient tells you what they are willing to accept in relation to their care and treatment.
- *Written*: Usually in the form of a formal consent document. Written consent is usually obtained when the procedure is invasive (surgery) or carries significant risk (immunisation).

Whilst a signed consent form demonstrates some evidence that the individual is agreeing to receive the treatment, Lord Donaldson, in Re T (Adult: Refusal of Treatment) (1992) (cited in Griffith and Tengnah 2008, p. 80) highlighted that 'the consent form is only as useful as the understanding of the person signing it'. It is important to ensure that accurate records are kept of how the consent was obtained.

When obtaining consent it is essential that the person is given an explanation of the treatment and any relevant facts such as risks and options in a manner that ensures understanding. Therefore, the health care professional making an assessment of the patient's capacity to consent for treatment must also assess the patient's ability to comprehend the information presented. (*More detail on how to do this and how it should be documented are addressed in other sections of this chapter.*)

Implied consent

Permission to provide treatment by the cooperation of the patient is described as 'implied consent'. For example, a patient rolling up their sleeve to have their blood pressure taken would imply that they are happy to have the procedure. Implied consent as defined by Griffith and Tengnah (2008) is 'the permission implied through the actions of the patient to a request to provide treatment'. However, acquiescence, where the person does not know what the procedure entails, is *not* consent. (*See further information on acquiescence in Chapter 3.*)

The law makes it clear that all health care professionals must give clear advice and information to the patient so that the patient can make a rational choice as to whether they are in agreement and give consent for the treatment or procedure to go ahead. There is a requirement to provide information that would be seen as what a reasonable body of equivalent health care professionals (e.g. level 1 state registered nurses) would have given in the same circumstances.

The fact that a patient attends a clinic or hospital does *not* imply that they are in agreement to be given treatment. In this case the person providing the procedure or treatment must ensure that the patient consents to the procedure prior to taking action.

Consent Case Study 3 – Tony

Tony has severe learning disabilities and requires a flu vaccine. Tony has limited speech. He attends the clinic for his flu vaccine with a support worker. Tony sits down in the treatment room with his support worker. The support worker takes Tony's coat off and rolls up his sleeve. This acquiescence does not necessarily mean that you can go ahead with the vaccination.

Before going ahead with administering the vaccine the health care professional needs to explain what is going to happen. This may require the use of pictures or demonstrating the equipment to be used. The health care professional needs to be sure that Tony has understood why he is there and what is going to happen before they proceed to give the vaccine.

If the health care professional does not believe that Tony has understood they then need to decide whether the vaccine needs to be given in his best interests. It may be decided that this vaccine cannot be given today and that Tony and his support worker need to go away and discuss this further.

Other factors to consider

Obtaining consent is such an important issue that it is worth taking time and considering the fullest range of factors that may influence the decision-making process. For some individuals the environment, time, venue and who they are with will have a significant impact on how they are able to process the information given to them and communicate their wants and wishes. (*You will find more guidance in Chapter 3 to help you support communication needs.*)

There are some general principles for deciding how to ensure you are providing the best opportunity to the patient in their decision making, described in the MCA 2005 code of practice. The code (p. 45) suggests that the following questions may help with this process:

- Does the person have a general understanding of what the decision they need to make and why they need to make it?
- Do they understand the consequences of making, or not making, the decision, or of deciding one way or another?
- Are they able to understand the information relevant to the decision?
- Can they weigh up the relative importance of the information?
- Can they use and retain the information as part of the decision-making process?
- Can they communicate their decision?

Reflective Learning Point:

Think about your own area of work – What would be a best practice approach to obtaining consent from a person with a learning disability?

Who is the decision maker?

When obtaining consent, if a patient has capacity the health care professional is bound by their decision, even where this could lead to their death. Where a person is not considered to have the capacity to make their own decisions, a key question to consider is '*Who is the decision maker*'?

The MCA 2005 tells us that many different people may be the decision maker. The person making the decision on behalf of the person who lacks capacity is known throughout the code as the 'decision maker'.

The following factors need to be taken into consideration:

- The person delivering the care is the decision maker.
- The decision maker varies depending on the individual's circumstances and the type of care or treatment being proposed, for example the surgeon when surgery is proposed; the social worker when a change of accommodation is proposed.
- Health and social care staff, family and unpaid carers can be decision makers.

Some health care professionals may feel particularly vulnerable when they are asked to make decisions regarding consent. Mencap (2002, p. 3) suggests that people who know the person well can help with this process by providing information that is relevant to the decision making, and also advise on the individual's preferences and choices. They recommend that the doctor should consult with family, friends, independent advocates and paid carers, and that every effort should be made to reach a consensus between relatives, carers and health professionals.

The decision maker is required to consider:

(a) The person's past and present wishes and feelings
(b) The beliefs and values that would influence his decision if he had capacity
(c) The other factors that he would consider if he was able to do so

The MCA code (2007, p. 90) suggests several options for when someone wants to challenge a decision maker's conclusions:

- Involve an advocate
- Get a second opinion
- Hold a formal or informal 'best interests' conference
- Attempt some form of mediation
- Pursue a complaint through the organisation's formal procedures

Where agreement still cannot be reached it may be necessary to refer the case to the courts to decide what is in the person's best interests.

Determining best interests

The MCA 2005 makes it clear that, when determining what is in a person's best interest, you must not make assumptions based on their condition – including in this case their learning disability. The following factors are important in determining best interests:

- Avoid making assumptions based on the person's age, appearance, condition or behaviour
- Consider a person's own wishes, feelings beliefs and values and any written statements made by the person when they had capacity
- Take account of the views of the family and informal carers
- Can the decision be put off until the person regains capacity
- Make every effort to involve the person in the decision-making process
- Demonstrate that you have carefully assessed any conflicting evidence or views
- Provide clear, objective reasons as to why you are acting in the person's best interest
- Take account of the views of any IMCA
- Take the less restrictive alternative or action

Section 5(1) of the MCA 2005 states that health care professionals have statutory or legal protection for acts of care and treatment providing they can demonstrate that they:

- Have taken reasonable steps to assess capacity to make a decision
- Reasonably believe that the person lacks capacity to make a decision
- Reasonably believe that the decision is in the person's best interest

Actions that might be covered by Section 5 include:

Personal care:

- Washing, dressing, personal hygiene, feeding
- Helping with communication
- Helping with mobility
- Helping someone take part in leisure activities
- Going into a person's home to check they are OK
- Doing someone's shopping or using their money
- Providing services into the home

Health care:

- Carrying out diagnostic procedures
- Providing emergency medical treatment
- Administering medication
- Providing nursing care
- Carrying out other medical procedures, for example taking blood

---

Consent Case Study 4 – Louise

Louise is 36 years old; she has severe learning disabilities. She has been displaying some unusual behaviours over the past month. She has been smacking her face and biting her wrist. Her care staff have noticed that she has had some rectal bleeding. She has seen the doctor and he would like her to have a rectal examination. He decides that she is unable to consent to the examination.

Her care staff are concerned that she will not cooperate with an investigation as she will not allow them to help her with any personal care. As rectal bleeding may indicate an underlying medical problem the doctor decides that it would be in her best interest to have a flexible sigmoidoscopy under sedation.

In this situation it is clear that the investigation is required and that as Louise is unable to consent, the doctor should discuss how he is going to proceed with the carers, next of kin, or relevant advocate, before going ahead. He may choose to provide some accessible information to help the carers and could also involve a learning disability liaison nurse to provide Louise and her care staff with support to prepare and plan for the hospital admission.

Mencap (2002) states that 'Morally speaking the "best interests" of a patient are served when their inherent dignity as a human being is observed and upheld.'

Where a health care professional acts in connection with the care and treatment of a person, and can demonstrate they have formed the reasonable belief that the individual lacks capacity, they can be confident they will not face civil liability or criminal prosecution if they act in the person's best interest.

However, health care professionals will *not* be protected if they act negligently. Actions only receive protection from liability if the Mental Capacity Acts' principles of best interest are followed.

Summary of best interests

- Establish who is the decision maker
- Consider all relevant circumstances as defined in Section 4(11) of the MCA
- Encourage participation from all relevant parties
- Ascertain whenever possible the person's feelings, beliefs and wishes
- Special consideration to be given for life-sustaining treatment

Quality of life considerations

Best interests are not just based on what would be of medical importance. Factors relating to social, psychological, spiritual and quality of life must also be taken into consideration. But what counts as quality of life and how is it measured?

The British Medical Association (BMA; 1999) guidance states that the term 'quality of life' is ambivalent and difficult to define. Mencap (2002) suggests that 'An individual's quality of life can never be solely judged in terms of "good health", "material wealth" or "long life", but must make account of their perceived values'.

It is important that we do not project our own values, beliefs and perspectives about disability onto a person with learning and/or physical disability. Their experience is very different from our own and therefore we cannot make a fair judgement of what is worthy life. Every individual has the same and equal right of access to medical treatment.

It is vital that health care professionals base their decision on whether to treat a person with a learning disability purely on the basis of their health need. The BMA guidelines make clear: 'It must always be clear that the doctor's role is not to assess the value or worth of the patient but that of the treatment'. Clinical decisions must always take the priority and treatment is not conditional on subjective quality of life measures.

The decision to withhold or impose medical treatment and care can be complex, even in relatively unproblematic cases. When the person has a learning disability and/or multiple physical disabilities that may prevent them from expressing a clear opinion on their treatment, decisions about what is in the person's best interest, based on maintaining or improving quality of life, become the responsibility of those providing treatment care and support.

Any decision to impose or withdraw treatment must be based on a comprehensive assessment of what is in the patient's best interests. It is essential that health care professionals making these decisions involve people who know the patient well as they can provide important information that may be relevant to the decision needing to be made.

There is no reason to assume that people with a learning disability (even if this is severe/profound) enjoy their lives any less than a person without a learning disability. They may appreciate different, though no less-valued life experiences, and health care professionals must attempt to understand 'how they experience the world'. This issue is demonstrated in the following case study.

Consent Case Study 5 – Gina

Gina is not independent in any aspect of self-care and she simply does not relate to television, cinema or theatre. However, she takes delight in her limited mobility by travelling in her wheelchair or car, finds enjoyment in food and drink and responds positively to friendly company. Often she giggles and sometimes erupts into fits of laughter for no obvious reason, but for the fact that she finds something funny or enjoyable in her own personal world.

Mencap (2002)

Settling disputes about best interests and quality of life

As in most aspects of life, disputes and differences in professional opinion may arise when making decisions about health interventions for people with a learning disability. The disputes could be about the decision made, best interests or quality-of-life issues.

If someone wishes to dispute a decision maker's conclusion, there are the following options:

1. Involve an advocate
2. Get a second opinion
3. Hold a best interest case conference
4. Attempt some form of mediation
5. Pursue a complaint though the organisation's formal procedures.

If attempts to resolve the dispute fail, the Court of Protection might ultimately need to decide what is in the person's best interests.

Mencap (2002) suggests the following guidelines will uphold the rights and interests of people with a learning disability:

1. A person with profound and multiple learning disabilities does not have a lower quality of life than a non-disabled person.
2. People with profound and multiple learning disabilities must have the same entitlement to medical treatment as anyone else. The existence of a learning disability does not justify different standards of medical treatment.
3. If quality of life criteria are relevant they should be applied to a person with a learning disability in the same manner as to a person without a disability. People may value and enjoy living a life we would not choose for ourselves. Considerations of quality of life are only relevant in the context of the gravity of illness and do not concern the degree or nature of a person's disability.
4. A decision to withhold treatment may be justifiable on the grounds that the treatment would lead to pain and suffering which is disproportionate to any benefit.
5. In any judgement of quality of life, doctors should compare the condition of the individual before the treatment with the expected condition after the treatment.
6. A comprehensive approach to the assessment of the quality of life of people with profound and multiple learning disabilities should be adopted from the perspective of the disabled person.
7. In circumstances where it is uncertain that medical treatment would be of benefit to patient with a learning disability, the patient's disability should not provide the grounds on which treatment is withheld.
8. Health care professionals must provide the patient and their family and carers with full and accurate information about the options for medical treatment and implications of treatment and non-treatment.

ADVOCACY AND EMPOWERMENT

An advocate is someone who acts on behalf of another and has their best interests in mind. This can be an informal or formal arrangement, and an advocate can be someone who is previously known to the person or not.

Empowerment for people with a learning disability means that they are actively involved, and have control where possible, in decisions taken in matters relating to themselves. In the context of general hospital care for people with a learning disability, this means empowering adults with a learning disability to make informed decisions about their health care, and providing the support that each individual with capacity requires to enable this to happen.

Independent mental capacity advocate

The aim of the IMCA service is to provide independent safeguards for people who lack capacity to make important decisions. An IMCA can provide support for a person who lacks capacity, and represent the individual's wishes in the decision-making process.

An IMCA will be instructed and consulted when *all* of the four following criteria are met:

1. The person lacks capacity
2. *Mandatory involvement* (except in cases of urgency):
   - An NHS body is proposing to provide, withhold or stop serious medical treatment
   - An NHS body is proposing to arrange accommodation or (change of accommodation) for a period of longer than 28 days or a stay in a care home for longer than 8 weeks
   - A local authority is proposing to arrange residential accommodation for a period longer than 8 weeks

   Discretionary involvement:
   - An NHS body or local authority has arranged accommodation and it is being reviewed
   - The person is subject to protective measures in adult protection cases, as either the victim or perpetrator
3. The person has no family or friends who are available and appropriate to support or represent them apart from professionals or paid workers providing care or treatment and has not previously named someone who could help with the decision and has not made an EPA or an LPA, or has a court-appointed deputy (other than solely to deal with their property and affairs).
4. The Mental Health Act 1983 does not apply to the decision. That is:
   - The treatment is not serious treatment for mental disorder that can be given without the person's consent
   - The accommodation is not required under the Mental Health Act by compulsory admission to hospital for 28 days or more.

When decisions about serious medical treatment are being considered for a person who lacks capacity and who does not have anyone appropriate to consult on their behalf, the health professional has a *duty* to instruct an IMCA, in accordance with Section 37 of the MCA 2005.

Chapter 10 of the MCA 2005 code of practice (2007) gives further detail about the IMCA service and how it works.

Chaperones

In some situations it may be appropriate to consider the use of a chaperone. Griffith and Tengnah (2008, p. 75) provide the following definitions of a chaperone:

- A chaperone provides a safeguard for a patient against humiliation, pain or distress during an examination and protects against verbal, physical sexual or other abuse.
- A chaperone provides physical and emotional comfort and reassurance to a patient during sensitive and intimate examinations or treatment.
- An experienced chaperone will identify unusual or unacceptable behaviour on the part of the health care professional.
- A chaperone may also provide protection for the health care professional against potentially abusive patients.

They explain that 'the chaperone's role may be passive, as a simple witness to the examination, or active, as someone who participates in the procedure by providing comfort and reassurance, and is skilled in identifying unacceptable behaviour'.

The Ayling Inquiry (Department of Health 2004), cited in Griffith and Tengnah (2008, p. 76), recommended that each NHS Trust has a chaperone policy and that best practice for a chaperone policy must ensure that:

- No family member or friend of a patient should be expected to undertake the chaperoning role.
- The presence of a chaperone during a clinical examination and treatment must be the clearly expressed choice of a patient.
- The patient must have the right to decline any chaperone offered if they so wish.
- Chaperoning should not be undertaken by other than trained staff: the use of untrained administrative staff as chaperones is not acceptable.

PLANNING FOR FUTURE CARE

People have a right to consent or refuse treatment, and a decision can be made in advance to refuse treatment in the future if they lose capacity.

Advanced decisions to refuse treatment

An advanced decision enables someone with capacity aged 18 or more, to make a decision about a time in the future when they may lack capacity. If a decision exists, health care professionals must follow this decision if it is valid and applicable in the current circumstances.

- An advanced decision is prepared when a person has capacity and will only apply at a time when they lack capacity to consent or refuse treatment.
- It must state precisely what treatment is to be refused and the circumstances when this may apply.
- Advanced decision to refuse treatment can be verbal or in writing and is binding.
- Advanced decisions regarding life-sustaining treatment must be in writing, signed and witnessed.

- An advanced decision can be withdrawn, by the individual while they have capacity, or by the decision maker if there is now a treatment that was not available at the time of the advance decision, or if the individual does something that is clearly inconsistent with the advance decision.
- Statements of views and wishes are important but not legally binding as an advanced decision.

It is important that health care professionals keep accurate notes where any verbal or written advanced decisions are received, to prevent any confusion in the future.

For further information, see MCA 2005, Sections 24–27; MCA code of practice (2007), Chapter 9).

EMERGENCY SITUATIONS

When a patient who lacks capacity is brought to the emergency department and requires emergency treatment to save life it will, in almost all cases, be necessary to provide treatment to the patient in the patient's best interests without delay. Attention, however, must again be made to any knowledge that the person has a valid advanced decision to refuse treatment (see earlier notes in 'planning for future care').

When an adult patient is admitted who may be temporarily unable to give consent, for example due to being unconscious, treatment required in order to preserve life may be given without their consent. However, where the treatment is not deemed urgent or life saving the health care professional must consider what steps are 'reasonable' in that particular case. It may be that the intervention can be delayed until the person can give consent. (*See also previous sections on capacity and obtaining consent.*)

As previously mentioned, Section 5(1) of the MCA 2005 provides possible protection for all actions carried out in connection with care or treatment on behalf of a patient who lacks capacity so long as it is shown that the health care professional acted in the patient's best interests.

WHAT TO DO WHEN CONSENT IS REFUSED

If an adult who has capacity makes a voluntary and appropriately informed decision to refuse proposed treatment then this decision must be respected. Legally, a competent adult can refuse consent to treatment, even when that refusal may result in harm or even death. It must also be recognised that the patient can withdraw their consent at any time including whilst the treatment is in progress.

There are exceptions to this with regard to patients who are subject to a section of the Mental Heath Act (MHA; 1993). Though there is no reason to assume a person lacks capacity because they are subject to a section of the MHA, health care professionals may consider using the MHA to detain and treat someone who lacks capacity to consent to treatment. (Chapter 13 of the MCA 2005 code of practice (2007) provides further advice on the relationship between the MCA and the Mental Health Act.)

Some patients may have an *advanced directive* that specifies their wishes with regard to treatment if they are in a situation where they become incapacitated and unable to express their wishes. An advanced decision to refuse treatment, made in advance while the person still has capacity, is outlined in more detail in Section 24(1) of the MCA 2005.

Therefore, if a health care professional is informed that the patient has an advanced decision regarding their treatment, they must consider the advanced decision as part of their assessment, ensuring that the advanced decision is valid and applicable to the proposed treatment.

For more information about advanced decisions, refer to Chapter 9 of the MCA 2005 code of practice (2007).

When a person is assessed as lacking capacity (in accordance with the five core principles described at the start of this chapter and the two-stage capacity test), and refuses to receive treatment, the best interest principles apply. Section 5 of the MCA 2005 permits the use of restraint when it is necessary to provide treatment. However, the level of restraint must be proportionate to the level of harm that the patient will experience if treatment is withheld.

In these cases the health care professional must consider whether the patient is being deprived of their liberty for the treatment to be completed. In hospital settings the identified need to deprive the patient of their liberty must be authorised by their supervisory body, for example the primary care trust/local authority.

Use of restraint and deprivation of liberty

The MCA code (2007, p. 284) defines deprivation of liberty as 'a term used in the European Convention on Human Rights about circumstances when a person's freedom is taken away'. It also defines restraint (p. 290) as 'The use or threat of force to help carry out an act that the person resists, or the restriction of a person's liberty of movement whether or not they resist'. This may include something as simple as holding a person's arm still to take a blood sample.

The criteria that may justify use of restraint are:

- The person lacks capacity in relation to the matter in question and it will be in the person's best interests for the act to be done.
- It is reasonable to believe that it is necessary to restrain the person to prevent harm to them.
- The restraint is a proportionate response to the likelihood of the person suffering from harm and the seriousness of that harm.

Staff are instructed only the minimum of force may be used for the shortest possible time. It is the responsibility of the person carrying out the restraint, or authorising it, to identify the reasons which justify it, for example the person would suffer harm unless they were restrained in some way.

Restraint, as allowed for in the MCA, permits the restriction of a person's liberty of movement if certain criteria are met. However, it does not permit any act that deprives a person of their liberty within the meaning of Article 5(1) of the European Convention on Human Rights, which states that 'everyone has a right to liberty and security of person'.

Restraint is permitted only in certain circumstances (Section 6(4) MCA 2005):

- It cannot conflict with decisions made by an attorney under an LPA or a court-appointed deputy.
- It cannot contradict a valid advanced refusal of treatment of which the provider was aware.
- It is reasonably believed that the action is necessary to prevent harm to the person.
- The act is proportionate response to the likelihood of the person suffering from harm, and the seriousness of that harm.

- Proportionate means the minimum necessary to achieve the desired outcome.
- 'Restraint' includes the use of or threat of use of force to secure an act that is resisted, or restriction of a person's liberty of movement (whether or not the person resists).
- 'Restraint' does not include subjecting the person to a deprivation of liberty within the meaning of Article 5(1) of the European convention of human rights.

The criteria that may justify the use of restraint are:

- The person lacks capacity in relation to the matter in question and it will be in the person's best interests for the act to be done.
- It is reasonable to believe that it is necessary to restrain the person to prevent harm to them.
- The restraint is a proportionate response to the likelihood of the person suffering from harm and the seriousness of that harm.

The Deprivation of Liberty Safeguards

The MCA 2005 provides a statutory framework for acting and making decisions in a person's best interest when the person lacks capacity to make those decisions for themselves.

Griffith and Tengnah (2008, p. 89) explain that 'There may be occasions when a person who lacks decision-making capacity is deprived of their liberty in their best interests when in hospital. To ensure that their human rights are respected, the deprivation of liberty must be authorised through an assessment by two health and social care professionals, including mental health nurses'. 'Where assessment agrees that the person should be deprived of their liberty in their best interests, this can be authorised for any period up to 12 months. A representative will be appointed who can ask for the issue to be reviewed'.

Depriving a person of their liberty may be necessary in some cases in providing effective care or treatment, but this decision *must* be made lawfully. Where care may involve depriving the person of their liberty during the care or treatment that is being proposed in the patient's best interest, safeguards have been introduced from April 2009 to protect those persons' rights and ensure that the treatment or care is in the persons' best interest.

The Deprivation of Liberty Safeguards provide legal protection for vulnerable people who may be deprived of their liberty in hospital or care homes. The safeguards do not apply to people who are detained under the Mental Health Act 1983. If patient care requires them to be deprived of their liberty then the hospital or care home *must* seek authorisation from a supervisory body in order to deprive the person of their liberty. A supervisory body is responsible for considering the requests for authorisations, commissioning the required assessments and, where the assessment agrees that the request for deprivation of liberty is in the person's best interest, authorising the deprivation of liberty.

Where the Deprivation of Liberty Safeguards are applied to a person in a hospital setting, the supervisory body can be established by accessing the following Department of Health website: http://www.dh.gov.uk/en/Publicationsandstatistics/Publications/PublicationsPolicy AndGuidance/DH_078466.

Depriving a person of their liberty is a serious matter and the decision needs to be very clearly documented in the patient notes with reference to the need for the treatment and how the decision to deprive the person of their liberty was made. The care plan must indicate what action will need to be taken and the duration of that action.

Deprivation of liberty can only be authorised if:

- It is in the patient's best interest to be protected from harm
- That the response is proportionate to the likelihood and seriousness of the harm
- There is no other less restrictive option

Consent Case Study 6 – Jason

Jason has severe learning disabilities and cerebral palsy and has been admitted to hospital for treatment due to collapsing at home. It is found that he has diabetes and there is evidence of renal hypotension and dehydration. Initially, Jason was compliant with care due to him being unwell; however, he soon regains awareness and pulls his cannula out preventing treatment required to maintain his blood sugar and hydration. Jason tries to get out of bed and has fallen on the floor.

Even with the support of his parents Jason is non-compliant with his treatment. The responsible doctor alongside the nursing staff and Jason's parents agree that it is in Jason's best interest to have the treatment. It is felt that the only option to ensure that Jason receives his treatment is to hold the cannula in place with a bandage so that he cannot remove it and to give him a mild sedative that will help to minimise the anxiety he is experiencing. It is also agreed that cot sides be in situ to prevent him from falling out of bed.

For further guidance on the application of the Deprivation of Liberty Safeguards see 'Deprivation of Liberty Safeguards, Code of Practice to supplement the main Mental Capacity Act 2005 Code of Practice (2009)'.

This can be downloaded from www.publicguardian.gov.uk or can be ordered from The Stationery Office.

RECORD KEEPING

Recording consent and capacity assessments in the patient's notes will provide evidence for staff if they face any challenges to their decision making and actions. The notes will help them to demonstrate that they had reasonable belief that the person lacked capacity and that the actions were in the person's best interest. Any refusal to consent must also be clearly recorded in the patient records.

To ensure this the record must show:

- What decision was to be made regarding capacity
- Why the decision was made
- How the decision was made, including evidence of how the patient was informed and any others involved in the process
- Why the decision is in the person's best interests

The record should be clearly identifiable in the patient's notes. It must be made clear that the assessment of capacity is in relation to a specific decision and that future assessment will be required for any other unrelated decision making. However, for health care assistants and support staff, helping patients to make daily decisions about their care who have previously been assessed as lacking capacity to make day-to-day decisions, need no formal assessment procedure or record.

Consent Case Study 7 – Lee

Lee has severe learning disabilities and is unable to verbally communicate his needs. He is known to have food preferences which are noted in his personal file. His care plan identifies that Lee is unable to make choices from the menu and that he will be assisted by the staff to complete the menu sheet. He also needs assistance to eat his food. It is sufficient for the health care assistant to document that 'Lee was given assistance to choose and to eat his meal'.

Lee is also unable to make decisions about his medication although he will take his medication as prescribed. Lee is unable to inform the staff when he needs to take pain medication.

Lee's care plan should include a pain profile (see pain profile in Chapter 4). This will inform staff how to identify when pain relief is required. The care plan must also make reference to the capacity assessment. The medication then can be administered as prescribed by the doctor. The nurse will then document in the case file that 'Lee was biting his hand which suggests that he is in pain. Pain relief was administered as prescribed'.

This case study demonstrates the importance of recording accurately all actions taken and the rationale for them.

CONCLUSION

This chapter explores the consent process from the perspective of a patient who has learning disabilities. It provides detailed information about consent and about how health care professional go about obtaining consent. It highlights the fact that consent from the patient is required for all health care interventions and also the fact that in most instances, with support, a person with a learning disability can give their own consent to treatment. This may include the use of an advocate or developing creative ways of empowering the person to make their own decisions.

Situations where there may be questions about the capacity of an individual to give consent are discussed, with guidance provided on assessing capacity and when to identify the potential for involving other professionals. Best practice guidance is given on how to obtain consent from a person with a learning disability, and an explanation of the legal framework that addresses consent is provided to support this guidance. This also includes advice for health care professionals on what to do when consent is refused, and how to make decisions based on the best interests of the individual.

Summary of Key Learning Points

The key learning points are:
- It is important to establish the presence of a learning disability early in the health care process – this can help you to identify any potential issues around obtaining or giving consent.
- People with learning disabilities have as much right to make decisions for themselves as anyone else.

- The health care professional must always be satisfied that the patient is consenting before proceeding with providing health care.
- For this consent to be valid the patient must:
  - Be competent to make that decision
  - Have received sufficient information to make the decision
  - Not be acting under duress
- Health care professionals need to be aware of the guidance in the MCA 2005 which provides a clear legal framework for consent and capacity to consent.
- The health care professional delivering care is the 'decision maker' when making decisions on behalf of a person who lacks capacity.
- The decision maker varies depending on the individual's circumstances and the type of care or treatment being proposed.
- Health services are required to make 'reasonable adjustments' to enable people with a learning disability to access the health care they need – this includes helping them to make informed choices about consent to treatment.

Links to KSF Competencies – Chapter 5

| | Level descriptors | | | |
	1	2	3	4
Core dimensions				
1 – Communication	Communicate with a limited range of people on day-to-day matters	Communicate with a range of people on a range of matters	Develop and maintain communication with people about difficult matters and/or in difficult situations	Develop and maintain communication with people on complex matters, issues and ideas and/or in complex situations
2 – Personal and people development	Contribute to own personal development	Develop own skills and knowledge and provide information to others to help their development	Develop oneself and contribute to the development of others	Develop oneself and others in areas of practice
3 – Health safety and security	Assist in maintaining own and others' health, safety and security	Monitor and maintain health, safety and security of self and others	Promote, monitor and maintain best practice in health, safety and security	Maintain and develop an environment and culture that improves health, safety and security
4 – Service improvement	Make changes in own practice and offer suggestions for improving services	Contribute to the improvement of services	Appraise, interpret and apply suggestions, recommendations and directives to improve services	Work in partnership with others to develop, take forward and evaluate direction, policies and strategies
5 – Quality	Maintain the quality of own work	Maintain quality in own work and encourage others to do so	Contribute to improving quality	Develop a culture that improves quality

6 – Equality and diversity	Act in ways that support equality and value diversity	Support equality and value diversity	Promote equality and value diversity	Develop a culture that promotes equality and values diversity

Health and well-being

HWB1 – Promotion of health and well-being and prevention of adverse effects on health and well-being	Contribute to promoting health and well-being and preventing adverse effects on health and well-being	Plan, develop and implement approaches to promote health and well-being and prevent adverse effects on health and well-being	Plan, develop and implement programmes to promote health and well-being and prevent adverse effects on health and well-being	Promote health and well-being and prevent adverse effects on health and well-being through contributing to the development, implementation and evaluation of related policies
HWB2 – Assessment and care planning to meet health and well-being needs	Assist in the assessment of people's health and well-being needs	Contribute to assessing health and well-being needs and planning how to meet those needs	Assess health and well-being needs and develop, monitor and review care plans to meet specific needs	Assess complex health and well-being needs and develop, monitor and review care plans to meet those needs
HWB3 – Protection of health and well-being	Recognise and report situations where there might be a need for protection	Contribute to protecting people at risk	Implement aspects of a protection plan and review its effectiveness	Develop and lead on the implementation of an overall protection plan
HWB4 – Enablement to address health and well-being needs	Help people meet daily health and well-being needs	Enable people to meet ongoing health and well-being needs	Enable people to address specific needs in relation to health and well-being	Empower people to realise and maintain their potential in relation to health and well-being
HWB5 – Provision of care to meet health and well-being needs	Undertake care activities to meet individuals' health and well-being needs	Undertake care activities to meet the health and well-being needs of individuals with a greater degree of dependency	Plan, deliver and evaluate care to meet people's health and well-being needs	Plan, deliver and evaluate care to address people's complex health and well-being needs
HWB6 – Assessment and treatment planning	Undertake tasks related to the assessment of physiological and psychological functioning	Contribute to the assessment of physiological and psychological functioning	Assess physiological and psychological functioning and develop, monitor and review related treatment plans	Assess physiological and psychological functioning when there are complex and/or undifferentiated abnormalities, diseases and disorders and develop, monitor and review related treatment plans

HWB7 – Interventions and treatments	Assist in providing interventions and/or treatments	Contribute to planning, delivering and monitoring interventions and/or treatments	Plan, deliver and evaluate interventions and/or treatments	Plan, deliver and evaluate interventions and/or treatments when there are complex issues and/or serious illness

Department of Health (2004). Reproduced under the terms of the Click-Use Licence.

REFERENCES

Beauchamp T and Childress J (1989) *Principles of Biomedical Ethics*. Oxford University Press, Oxford.

British Medical Association (1999) *Withholding and Withdrawing Life-Prolonging Medical Treatment. Guidance for Decision Making*. BMJ Books, London.

Department for Constitutional Affairs (2005) *Mental Capacity Act 2005*. The Stationary Office, London.

Department for Constitutional Affairs (2007) *Mental Capacity Act 2005 – Code of Practice*. The Stationary Office, London.

Department of Health (1995) *Disability Discrimination Act*. HMSO, London.

Department of Health (1998) *Human Rights Act*. HMSO, London.

Department of Health (DH) (1999) *Code of Practice to the Mental Health Act 1983*. HMSO, London.

Department of Health (2004) *The NHS Knowledge and Skills Framework (NHS KSF) and the Development Review Process. Appendix 1: Overview of the NHS KSF*. HMSO, London.

Department of Health (2005) *Disability Discrimination Act*. HMSO, London.

Enduring Powers of Attorney Act (1985) HMSO, London.

Griffith R and Tengnah C (2008) *Law and Professional Issues in Nursing*. Learning Matters Ltd., Exeter.

Mencap (2002) *'Quality of Life' and Medical Decision Making for Adults with Profound and Multiple Learning Disabilities*. Mencap, London.

Ministry of Justice (2008) *Deprivation of Liberty Safeguards. Code of Practice to Supplement the Main Mental Capacity Act 2005 Code of Practice*. HMSO, London.

Nursing and Midwifery Council (NMC) (2008) *The Code: Standards of Conduct, Performance and Ethics for Nurses and Midwives*. NMC, London.

Nursing and Midwifery Council (NMC) (2009) Decisions, decisions. *NMC News*, February.

Royal College of Nursing (RCN) (2006) *Meeting the Health Needs of People with Learning Disabilities*. RCN, London.

Scottish Executive (2000) *Adults with Incapacity Act*. NHSS, Edinburgh.

6 Ethical and Political Aspects of Care

INTRODUCTION

This chapter explores the ethical and political aspects of health care and how they influence the care provided to people with a learning disability. The professional responsibility and accountability of all health care professionals is discussed, in particular their responsibilities for ethical decision making and the need to safeguard and protect vulnerable children and adults. The values and beliefs that underpin professional practice are explored and the issue of 'normalisation' is explained and its importance in ensuring health care professionals adapt the environment to meet the needs of the person with a learning disability within ordinary services.

The political issues and their influence on the way that services have been provided for people with a learning disability are outlined, and some of the key national policy documents are considered, including information about investigations into examples of poor practice. A brief outline is included of the different health care professionals who may be involved with people with a learning disability and their roles. This is intended to encourage partnership working through a better understanding of skills and competencies, and areas of work.

The chapter concludes with a consideration of what future services might look like and how we can best meet the health needs of people with a learning disability. This includes personal and organisational checklists and a benchmark for good practice in providing general hospital care for people with a learning disability.

HEALTH CARE ETHICS AND PROFESSIONAL ACCOUNTABILITY

Professional accountability

The Department of Health published 'The Statement of NHS Accountability' in January 2009, which provides a summary of the current structure and functions of the NHS in England. This document accompanies the NHS Constitution, which describes the system of roles and responsibilities, clarifies how the NHS works, and how it is accountable at a local and national level. It sets out principles to guide how all parts of the NHS should act and make decisions. The bodies with devolved responsibility for health care in Scotland, Wales and Northern Ireland have also signed up to a set of common principles and the principles of the NHS are recognised as the same across the United Kingdom (Department of Health 2009a, b).

General Hospital Care for People with Learning Disabilities, First Edition by Lynn Hannon and Julie Clift
© 2011 Blackwell Publishing Ltd

The NHS Constitution was one of the recommendations made by Lord Darzi in his report 'High Quality Care for All' which set out a 10-year plan to provide the highest quality of care and service for patients in England (Department of Health 2008). The NHS Constitution brings together for the first time what staff, patients and public can expect from the NHS and outlines the seven key principles that guide the NHS in all it does, illustrated in the box below:

Box 6.1   Principles that guide the NHS

1. The NHS provides a *comprehensive service* available to all, irrespective of gender, race, disability, age, religion or sexual orientation.
2. Access is based on *clinical need*, not on an individual's ability to pay.
3. The NHS aspires to *high standards* of excellence and professionalism in everything it does.
4. NHS services must reflect the *needs and preferences* of patients, their families and their carers – that is, involving and consulting them.
5. The NHS *works together* across organisations, in the interest of patients, local communities and the wider population.
6. The NHS is committed to providing *best value* for taxpayer's money and the most effective and fair use of finite resources.
7. The NHS is *rightly accountable* to the public, communities and patients that it serves – it takes most of its decisions locally and gives us the chance to influence and scrutinise its performance and priorities.

These principles are supported by a set of NHS values, which are outlined in Box 6.2:

Box 6.2   NHS Values

- Respect and dignity – valuing each person as an individual
- Commitment to quality of care
- Compassion
- Improving lives
- Working together for patients
- Everyone counts – making sure that nobody is excluded

The Constitution also includes four pledges to staff stating that the NHS will strive to:

1. Provide well-designed and rewarding jobs that make a difference to patients, their families, carers and communities
2. Provide personal development, access to appropriate training and line management support to succeed
3. Provide support and opportunities to keep people healthy and safe
4. Engage staff in decisions that affect them and the services they provide

The Statement of NHS Accountability continues to explain that the NHS is funded by national taxation with the government providing funds to the Department of Health to provide services. The Secretary of State for Health is accountable to Parliament and the general public for the promotion of a comprehensive health service and the use of public money. The NHS currently spends around £100 billion a year – equivalent to nearly £2,000 per person on average. The majority of this money is allocated directly to Primary Care Trusts who are responsible for commissioning services for their population.

The Statement of NHS Accountability states (p. 6) that 'All organisations that provide care for NHS patients are responsible for ensuring that their services meet appropriate levels of safety and quality'. It explains that all these organisations are held to account in two main ways:

1. By the local Primary Care Trust, which generally has the power to end the contract with the provider or to commission services from elsewhere; and
2. By the regulators (e.g. Strategic Health Authorities, Monitor, independent regulators)

It continues to explain that from April 2009 the **Care Quality Commission** will be the independent regulator for all health services. Their principal functions will be to:

*   Register health care providers (whether or not they provide services for the NHS)
*   Monitor compliance with registration requirements and, if necessary, use its enforcement powers to ensure all service providers meet those requirements
*   Review and publish comparative information on organisations providing and commissioning health care, and undertake reviews or studies of particular kinds of care
*   Monitor the operation of the Mental Health Act and Mental Capacity Act

All of these functions will have an impact on health care provided to people with a learning disability in general hospital settings.

Primary Care Trusts are responsible for improving the health and well-being of their local population working in partnership with other NHS trusts, and other agencies such as local authorities and voluntary/independent sector organisations. They do this by assessing health needs then commissioning services to meet those needs. Services commissioned include general practice, dental practice, community pharmacy and general hospital services.

Professional regulatory bodies are responsible for the regulation of every health care professional. For example, the General Medical Council regulates doctors, and the Nursing and Midwifery Council regulates nurses. Regulatory bodies ensure that all registered health care professionals are bound to act with regard to a professional code of conduct which sets out standards of practice and professional accountability. These codes, published and monitored by the relevant professional body, provide a framework for monitoring and evaluating professional practice, dealing with concerns about misconduct, ensuring standards are maintained and dealing with fitness to practice issues.

The General Medical Council (2001) (Good Medical Practice, paragraph 5) makes the following statement: 'Health care is increasingly provided by multi-disciplinary teams. Working in a team does not change your personal accountability for your professional conduct and the care you provide'.

Other specialist national bodies such as the National Institute for Clinical Excellence, and the Medicines and Healthcare Products Regulatory Agency provide advice on best practice and professional accountability at a national level.

The NHS is also accountable to patients who use its services and the general public, and has a legal duty to involve people who use health services, or their representatives, in decisions about those services. This includes active involvement in planning and providing services, developing new services or changing the way that services operate. This can even include becoming involved as a member of a foundation trust. Support would probably be needed to enable people with a learning disability to play an active part in this process but the value of the contribution would be high.

Local authorities operate two ways of enabling members of the public to contribute a voice to how local health services are planned and delivered:

- *Local Involvement Networks* (LINks) are made up of individuals and community groups who work together to improve local health and social care services.
- *Overview and Scrutiny Committees* have the power to scrutinise the operation and planning of local health services.

NHS trusts are legally obliged to allow LINks representative to enter and view their services. They are also required to respond to recommendations made by LINks and tell them what actions they will take in response to their recommendations.

Every organisation providing health care to people with a learning disability should have a local complaint procedure that should be made available to people (in an accessible format) when requested. This procedure should tell people how their complaint will be dealt with and also outline timescales for responding to complaints.

The Parliamentary and Health Service Ombudsman provides the highest level of accountability for complaints about health service provision. The Ombudsman is accountable to Parliament and is independent of the NHS. The Ombudsman conducts investigations into complaints where public bodies have not acted properly or fairly, or have provided a poor service.

The 2009 Ombudsman report into the deaths of six people with a learning disability whilst in hospital is explored later in this chapter.

Ethical decision making

Chaloner (2007) stated that 'Ethics is concerned with determining what is right and wrong with regards to our decisions and actions'. She explains how exploring ethical issue is a familiar process and as health professionals we participate in ethical decision making every day.

Reflective Learning Point:

The question 'Should I tell my friend what people are saying about him?' will demand consideration of the potential harms and benefits of such an action. I may decide I have a duty to tell him as this is the 'right thing to do'.

Chaloner (2007)

Chaloner continues to highlight the following basic ethical concepts:

Box 6.3   Basic Ethical Concepts

- *Avoiding harm*: Perhaps the most essential ethical concept. It is generally considered to be the basis for good practice.
- *Obligations and duties*: Identifying our moral obligations to other people can help us to determine what we should do in a given situation.
- *Assessing the consequences of actions*: The ethically appropriate action may be determined by calculating its potential benefits and harm.
- *Autonomy and rights*: Respect for autonomy and acknowledging individual rights provides a basis for respecting others.
- *Best interests*: Identifying and acting in the best interests of others often provides ethical justification for an action or decision.
- *Values and beliefs*: From these we formulate general ethical principles that provide guidance to decisions and actions.

Chaloner (2007), reproduced with kind permission of the RCN.

The General Medical Council (2001) (Good Medical Practice, paragraph 36) makes the following statement:

'The investigation and treatment you provide or arrange must be based on your clinical judgement of patients' needs and the likely effectiveness of treatment. You must not allow your views about a patient's lifestyle, culture, beliefs, race, colour, gender, sexuality, disability, age or social or economic status to prejudice the treatment you give'.

The Mental Capacity Act 2005 provides those supporting people with learning disabilities with the statutory framework for ethical decision making. It empowers those who have capacity to make their own decisions but, more importantly for those who lack capacity to make their own decisions and rely on others to make decisions for them, it provides a duty to ensure that those decisions are made in their best interests. (Chapter 5 discussed in detail how the Mental Capacity Act 2005 is implemented in practice.)

As practitioners there are times when we face the dilemma of withholding information that we believe may cause distress to the patient and potentially prevent the procedure going ahead. The dilemma that health care professionals face with regard to truth telling and deception are often due to the clashing of the ethical principles that are described in Chapter 5.

The principles of 'respect for autonomy' and 'non-malfeasance' cause conflict when deciding to withhold information that may cause distress. Though this is done with the intent to protect the patient, it does not respect the person's right to autonomy in decision making if the patient does not receive all the information they require to be able to make those decisions. For example, if it is decided by the health care team that giving a diagnosis of terminal cancer to the patient will cause depression and therefore psychological harm, it may be the team's decision not to tell the patient. This is often the case for people with learning disabilities. The family or carers in a wish to 'not upset' the person may request that the patient is not informed of the diagnosis.

Thompson et al. (2000) suggest that nurses' knowledge and status give them not only the power to help vulnerable people, but also power over such people. People with learning disabilities often face paternalistic support with regard to decision making in all aspects of their lives, and particularly when it is in relation to decision making about their health care. Deciding to withhold information, or only telling the patient part of the diagnosis or treatment, is often based on what the fear of the consequence to the patient is of being given the full picture.

Health care professionals can feel under pressure from family and carers to withhold information because of their fear of the outcome. However, the health care professional has a responsibility to respect that people with learning disabilities have the same rights as other patients and they should consider the patient's competence to decide whether or not their family or carer should be informed of their diagnosis and treatment, and be placed in the position to make these decisions for them.

The argument that deception is favourable needs to be rigorously explored in each specific case. It may be felt that if telling a patient that 'it won't hurt' so that they will not be worried about a blood test may be the right thing to say. However, if (as it may well do) the blood test does hurt, the patient is very unlikely to trust the next person who needs to take blood. As argued by Collis (2006), there are some who support the use of deception to protect patients particularly those with terminal diagnosis.

Collis also suggests that the use of deception with patients who have a compromised level of competency could be deemed more acceptable, especially where the use of covert administration of medication is required when it is the sole method of ensuring that medication required for their health is taken. (*See later section for further discussion of this issue.*)

The following statement is a view advocated by Whatt (2008).

'In a professional environment much respect is given to truth telling as an absolute but there is a certain simplicity in this which is not always fitting when caring for people with learning disabilities who lack capacity. There may be occasions when deception is therapeutically relevant'.

Ethical and Political Case Study 1 – Ethical Decision Making

Sajida has moderate learning disabilities and Down's syndrome. She was recently diagnosed with the early stages of dementia. It has been noticed that Sajida is having difficulty moving around her home especially at night and it is identified that she needs to have a cataract removed from her right eye.

When Sajida is told that she is going into hospital to have an operation on her eye she becomes distressed and says that she does not want to have an operation. Sajida's family are very concerned that she has the cataract removed and asks that she is not told that she is going to have an operation until the day she is due to be admitted to hospital and then she will be told that she is going to have a blood test. The family believe that if she is told she is going to hospital for the surgery she will refuse to attend.

As health care professionals we have a duty not to lie, deceive or coerce our patients in an attempt to gain their cooperation with care or treatment. The ethical principles of 'justice', 'beneficence', 'autonomy', and 'non-malfeasance' as described in Chapter 5 encourage us to ensure that our patients are treated without causing any harm and that they are able to make decisions for themselves based on accurate information. The Mental Capacity Act 2005 also requires that we provide information to patients, even if they are assessed as lacking capacity to make their own decisions, to help them understand what the treatment will entail.

In Sajida's situation, even though she is afraid of having surgery, possibly due to her lack of understanding of what this will entail, it would not be ethically sound not to inform her of what coming into hospital will entail.

Sajida would probably benefit from an accessible information document that outlines her treatment and admission to hospital. By preparing Sajida in this way you may help to reduce the level of anxiety she is experiencing regarding the procedure and her family and health care professionals will be able to assess how much she understands about the admission and treatment. They will then be able to decide how best to plan the admission and what support she will require to ensure that they are able to complete the treatment with the minimum of distress for Sajida. It may be decided that the use of the word 'operation' is what causes her the most distress but by saying she will have a 'procedure' lessens her anxiety.

It is essential that this type of decision making is based on a sound rationale and in taking into account the thoughts and feelings of family and carers the health care professional is protected from any legal and moral liability.

Reflective Learning Point:

Think of a situation in your own area of work where you have chosen to withhold information from a patient:

- What rationale did you use to make this decision?
- What factors influenced your decision?
- Did you act in the person's best interests?

Ethical and Political Case Study 2 – Ethical Decision Making

Martin has epilepsy and learning disabilities. Periodically he needs to have a blood test because he is prescribed anticonvulsant medication. Martin understands that he takes medication for his epilepsy but lacks capacity to understand why he needs to have his blood taken to test the anticonvulsant level. Martin does not like having blood taken but is usually compliant at the time. It is known that he becomes very upset to the point of self-harming by banging his forehead if he is aware that he needs to have blood taken.

It is decided that Martin will not be informed that he is going to have a blood test until a few minutes before the appointment time to avoid him having to experience the anxiety of waiting for the appointment.

This type of benevolent deceit may be judged to be in the best interest of the patient because the distress of knowing he is going for a blood test causes Martin to injure himself significantly by banging his head.

The decision to withhold information from a patient, or benevolent deceit in the form of withholding or manipulating the truth can be justifiable if in doing so the trust of the patient is not threatened. Consideration of the fact that if telling the truth will cause distress is seen as acceptable by some, as described by Whatt (2008). However, he adds that not everyone agrees with this assertion and that by hiding the truth the health care professional is taking a paternalistic protective stance that takes away the patient's rights to act autonomously.

The rationale for withholding selective information may rest on the ethical principle of 'non-malfeasance' and 'beneficence'. Whatt (2008) summarises this by saying 'Consequently, there may be occasions when it is considered ethically justifiable to deprive an individual of the absolute truth if the intention is to do good and/or prevent harm'. He continues to state, 'We must meticulously consider the potential to violate an individual's autonomy with the excuse of preventing harm'.

We should not disregard the patient's right to autonomy by deception just because the patient does not have the ability to act independently. Slevin (2009) reminds us that 'a person with a learning disability should have the autonomy to make life choices as any other person of a similar age can'. He continues, 'They also need to be empowered to make choices and a key role of a practitioner/carer is empowering individuals and groups to make choices'. Slevin stresses that most people can give consent if the information is provided in a way that they are able to understand and that it is unethical not to obtain consent from those with the least communication skills because not to do so could result in enforced treatment.

'Ethical Virtues' as described by Slevin incorporate the principles of truthfulness with compassion, caring, respecting others, fairness and justice, accepting others and treating people as equals.

Reflective Learning Point:

'No one should be exposed to care or treatment they do not consent to and carers should be guided in their practice by ethical virtues that show respect for clients as human beings'. Slevin (2009)

Harvey and Stobbart, cited in Gates (2005), recommend a *five-step* reflective process to ethical decision making especially when making decisions in partnership with others.

Step 1: how to decide if it is an ethical dilemma

As not all problems are ethical in nature a true ethical dilemma is identified when the moral values of the nurse and the client are vastly incongruent. In such a situation, the nurse through self-awareness should recognise the impact of her moral beliefs and values on the relationship with the client. It is essential to gather as much information as you can and by speaking to all those involved in the care of the individual, colleagues, family carers and as much as possible the person themselves. Not everyone's opinion will be the same and there may be no logical solution.

Step 2: identify and examine your own views and values on the issues

Consider the point of the issue that causes you the dilemma. Acknowledge that people can reach different conclusions. Discuss the issue in clinical supervision or as part of a multi-disciplinary forum or similar reflective environment.

Step 3: identify the problem

After reviewing the relevant information develop a clear statement of the problem. This statement forms the basis of the negotiation with others.

Step 4: gather all courses of potential actions and conflicts

Ensure that all the information and possible actions to resolve the dilemma are documented and this should be discussed in a multi-disciplinary forum.

Step 5: evaluate the actions taken

The care plan should have a clear date for review of the agreed actions. Documentation of the decision made and record of every step related to the ethical decision-making process. The care plan must be clear about how to measure the effectiveness of the decisions made.

Ethical and Political Case Study 3 – Ethical Dilemmas

Marie is 54 and requires a 'Whipple's resection'. This surgery is particularly high risk although the chance of her surviving without surgery is poor. Marie is informed that there is a chance that she may become diabetic after the surgery and becomes distressed about the possibility of having to inject insulin.

The Surgeon's dilemmas: Does this lady have capacity to make the decision to have surgery? Can she cope? Will she pull the tubes out in intensive care? Will she cooperate with the required treatment after surgery?

The acute liaison nurse provided accessible information for Marie to help her to understand the procedure and the process of her admission and post-operative treatment. The surgeon went ahead in her best interests deciding that Marie had a basic understanding of the procedure – not enough to be able to consent but enough so that she could be compliant and tolerate the surgery and treatment.

Ethical and Political Case Study 4 – Ethical Dilemmas

Bill is 62 and requires high-risk carotid artery surgery. Chances are he will die if he does not have the surgery but the surgery carries a high risk and he could die as a result of the surgery. The consultant was reluctant to proceed unless Bill could weigh up the risks and benefits of the surgery and the Surgeon was feeling that he can only go ahead if Bill has the capacity to make that decision.

The acute liaison nurse worked with Bill to explain the procedure and help him to understand the risks involved. Bill was able to reflect back what he had been told and expressed a wish to have the surgery. The acute liaison nurse was concerned that it was his fear of dying that was prompting him to have the surgery, and wondered whether he really understood that he could die anyway if he had the surgery.

Bill did have the surgery as the surgeon felt that Bill understood enough about the procedure to consent to his operation.

In both these cases it was concerns about the person having a learning disability and their ability to cope with difficult decision making and complex treatments that created the ethical dilemmas.

Reflective Learning Point:

Would we be put under such scrutiny before a surgeon agreed to carry out a necessary procedure for us?

Covert administration of medication

The Nursing and Midwifery Council (NMC 2007) recognises and gives advice with regard to the covert administration of medicines. A position statement in 2007 recognised the importance of respecting the autonomy of the patient and the right to refuse treatment, including taking prescribed medication. The NMC advises that in the exceptional cases where people lack the capacity to make the decision to take prescribed medication, and are refusing to take the medication on request, that the medication may be administered in food without the patient having knowledge that this is being done. (*See also the guidance on consent and best interests in Chapter 5.*)

Patients may have a variety of reasons for refusing medication and wherever possible the nurse should endeavour to establish a preferred method of administration, for example changing tablets to syrups or offering medication with a preferred drink or food. If covert administration is considered in the patient's best interest by the care team it must be clearly documented that:

- The patient lacks capacity
- The expectation is that the patient will benefit from the measure
- That all other options for administration have been tried
- The decision has been discussed with the next of kin or nominated representative
- That the pharmacy agrees that the medication can be effectively administered in the proposed method (e.g. the medication is crushable)
- The date for review
- The GP must be informed in writing

Ethical and Political Case Study 5 – Covert Administration of Medication

Alison has been admitted to hospital with acute cellulitis and requires antibiotics. She is refusing to take the medication because she says they make her feel sick.

The nurse establishes by talking with her support staff when they visit the ward that they have problems when Alison is prescribed any new medication.

She has experience reactions to medication in the past which has caused nausea and vomiting. When she has refused medication in the past they have given her medication with strawberry jam.

The nurse discusses the case with the ward doctor who makes the decision that Alison does not have capacity to understand the benefits of taking the medication she has been prescribed and that it is in her best interest to have the medication as suggested by her support staff.

> The GP is contacted who confirms that medication has been prescribed for cellulitis in the past and it has been agreed that it can be administered covertly by her care staff at home.
>
> Pharmacy is contacted and agrees that the medication can be administered in this way. The plan is documented in the medical notes.

SAFEGUARDING CHILDREN AND VULNERABLE ADULTS

The issue of safeguarding people with a learning disability and providing protection from abuse is a key aspect of ethical care. The potential for abuse is high, especially where people are dependent on another for full personal care needs. For many people the setting in which they live make them more vulnerable to abuse from family, carers and other service users. It is estimated that 5–10% of vulnerable adults suffer from some sort of abuse or neglect.

It is widely accepted that adults with learning disabilities are potential victims of abuse and neglect. This was highlighted in the Healthcare Commission's (2007a, b) reports into abuse in NHS learning disability services in Cornwall and Merton and Sutton. They are at increased risk as a result of their vulnerability, the lack of insight into what constitutes abuse, and an inability to communicate that they are experiencing abuse. As explored in Chapter 4, challenging behaviour may be the person's way of exhibiting that they are experiencing abuse.

Abuse is commonly experienced by adults with learning disabilities. The Department of Health and Home Office (2000) stresses the importance of early reporting and prompt investigation of any allegations of abuse. Therefore, it is vital to follow your organisation's policy on responding to and the reporting of suspected or actual abuse immediately.

Abuse as defined by the Department of Health and the Nursing and Midwifery Council is generalised as:

> 'Abuse is a violation of an individual's civil and human rights by another person or persons' (Department of Health 2000).
>
> 'Abuse within the practitioner–client relationship is the result of the misuse of power or a betrayal of trust, respect or intimacy between the practitioner and the client, which the practitioner should know would cause physical or emotional harm to the client' (NMC 2002).

These definitions therefore suggest that abuse occurs when one person exerts power over another. It is thought that people with learning disabilities are particularly vulnerable to abuse because they are often supported in situations where they are cared for and, due to a number of factors, are susceptible to abuse. McCartney and Campbell (cited in Jenkins and Davis 2004) suggest that people with a learning disability have a heightened risk of abuse because they may have additional challenges which include:

- *Communication deficits*: This is when the person is unable to verbally communicate effectively their wants and wishes and decisions may be made for them in the interest of the carer. Not being able to communicate abuse can lead to the person displaying challenging or unusual behaviour as a means to communicate their distress.

- *Challenging behaviour*: People who present challenges to their family or carers are at significant risk of harm as a result of poor management of the behaviour. Overuse of physical restraint may cause physical or emotional injury to manage physical aggression or the use of seclusion to prevent harm to others.
- *Physical health problems*: The stress of managing complex physical health needs can be demanding on carers thus leading to health needs being neglected or ignored.
- *The dependence on others* for intimate care needs.

Abuse may take a number of forms which fall into the following widely accepted categories:

Physical abuse

This is generally agreed to be hitting, punching, kicking, hair pulling but also includes over- or misuse of medication, undue or excessive use of restraint. Physical abuse can often be identified by the evidence of physical injury which may be noted during a physical examination or during personal care. Concerns may be raised if a person appears oversedated by their medication, or the over-exertion of physical restraint for health care procedures, or for example force feeding.

Financial abuse

This is commonly the theft or fraudulent use of a person's finances or possessions. This may be identifiable where carers are reluctant to purchase required items for care, for example continence aids.

Sexual abuse

This includes all sexual incidents such as rape and sexual assault. For people with learning disabilities the issue of consent to sexual activity often leads to concerns that the person has been subject to sexual abuse if they are unaware of the nature or consequences of the activity.

Psychological abuse

This is a more difficult form of abuse to define as it is a particularly subjective category. It may include issues such as harassment, bullying, denial of attention, denial of rights. This may be evident when the perpetrator appears to overrule the person's choices or decisions. You may notice that the person looks to the carer for reassurance before giving an answer to questions or may be reluctant to verbalise when the perpetrator is present when they would normally engage with the conversation.

Neglect

Neglect is the withholding of basic care resulting in physical harm such as malnutrition or poor personal hygiene. This may be in the form of passive neglect where there is a failure to ensure that the person has access to the health care they require.

It is concerning that abuse is known to be perpetrated on the whole by family members and carers. A study by Rushton and Beaumont (cited in Jenkins and Davis 2004) highlighted that 44% of family members and 24% of carers were identified as abusers, with another 15% being other vulnerable adults being the perpetrators of the abuse. The most common type of abuse was physical abuse which accounted for 50% of the cases researched.

Reflective Learning Point:

What kind of signs and symptoms might be an indication of abuse when seen in someone with a learning disability?

   Do you know what your organisation's policy is on how to respond to or report suspected or actual abuse?

Sexual boundaries

The Council for Healthcare Regulatory Excellence (2009) issued information for patients and carers titled 'Clear sexual boundaries between healthcare professionals and patients'. This document (p. 2) contains information about:

- What sexual boundaries are and why they are important
- The responsibility of health care professionals to establish and maintain clear sexual boundaries with patients and carers, and not to display sexualised behaviour towards them
- What you should do if you are concerned that a health care professional has breached sexual boundaries

   The document explains (p. 3) that 'a breach of sexual boundaries occurs when a healthcare professional displays sexualised behaviour towards you' and this is defined as 'acts, words or behaviour designed or intended to arouse or gratify sexual impulses or desires. Breaches of sexual boundaries do not just include criminal acts such as rape or sexual assault, but cover a range of behaviours including the use of sexual humour or innuendo, and making inappropriate comments about your body'. This can also include comments made in your presence even if they are not about you, and applies to both male and female health care workers.

   People with learning disability are particularly vulnerable to actions of this kind, especially if they have limited communication skills and are not able to explain this kind of behaviour to someone else. They may also not understand the nature of the behaviour and know that it is wrong raising further concerns about consent. It is the responsibility of health care professionals to establish and maintain clear sexual boundaries and this should also include always asking patients for permission before touching them. The health care professional is in a position of trust and has a duty to ensure the safety and well-being of their patients. A power imbalance can arise if clear boundaries are not maintained.

   Any sexualised behaviour observed by another health care professional should be reported immediately. This would usually be made to the responsible line manager/employer in the first instance though the seriousness of the behaviour may also mean that the police or local social services should be contacted directly. A report may also be made to the health care professional's regulatory body (e.g. General Medical Council). The normal complaint procedures within the organisation could also be used for this purpose.

   It is also important to acknowledge that this type of behaviour can sometimes be demonstrated by a patient towards the health care professional. This behaviour could mean that care is transferred to another professional. The guidance also explains (p. 7) that in the case of former patients a sexual relationship would almost never be appropriate if:

- The health care professional used a power imbalance or information gained about you while he or she was treating you
- The health care professional/patient relationship involved long-term emotional or psychological support
- The patient was suffering from mental health problems or a condition that affected their judgement at the time the health care professional was treating them

The document provides a list of useful appendices that outline examples of sexualised behaviour, contact details of support organisations and regulatory bodies, and a list of useful websites. Further information can be obtained from: www.chre.org.uk.

Criminal Record Bureau checks

Criminal Record Bureau (CRB) checks should be completed for all health care staff as part of standard pre-employment checking procedures and before individuals start in post. This is essential for all health professionals in line with the NHS Employment Check Standards (2008) and provides some assurance that only suitable people are employed in this kind of role.

The CRB provides access to information across England and Wales (with a similar scheme operating in Scotland) about criminal convictions and other police records. The information provided by the CRB is known as a 'Disclosure' and can help employers make an informed decision on whether or not to appoint a prospective employee.

There are currently two levels of check available for employment purposes:

- *Standard* – appropriate for posts involving access to patients in the course of normal duties (e.g. receptionist, domestic)
- *Enhanced* – appropriate for posts where in addition to having access to patients in the course of normal duties, the position must also involve 'regularly caring for, training, supervising or being in sole charge of persons aged under 18 or vulnerable adults' (e.g. nurse, allied health professional, health care worker)

Standard or enhanced checks are mandatory in the NHS for all staff who have regular contact with patients as part of their normal duties. All health care professionals providing direct care will require an enhanced CRB check. Employers cannot, by law, request a Disclosure for any position that is not identified as exempts from the Rehabilitation of Offenders Act (ROA) 1974 (Exceptions) Order 1975. All appointments covered by the ROA are subject to a criminal record check.

Possession of a criminal offence does not automatically make an applicant unsuitable for employment in the NHS. Organisations should have guidance available for the recruitment of ex-offenders and the suitability for employment will depend on the nature of the position.

Further information about CRB checks can be found at: www.crb.gov.uk.

Vetting and barring scheme

The Safeguarding Vulnerable Groups Act (2006) introduced a new vetting and barring scheme (VBS) to further enable the protection of children and vulnerable adults. The new VBS will be administered by the Independent Safeguarding Authority (ISA) and was launched in England, Wales and Northern Ireland on 12 October 2009. Following the change of Government in May 2010 the new coalition announced on 15 June 2010 that the whole ISA scheme was to be reviewed meaning that individual applications for registration onto the scheme will not begin until this review is completed.

The new scheme is a mandatory addition to the service currently provided by the CRB and does not replace a (CRB) Disclosure.

The VBS was developed in response to the Bichard Inquiry and introduces new measures for vetting people working or volunteering with children or vulnerable adults, and making decisions about who should be barred. The Safeguarding Vulnerable Groups Act (2006) defines the scope of the scheme and provides that certain activities in relation to vulnerable groups are regulated as follows:

Regulated Activity:
- Any activity of a *specified nature* that involves contact with children or vulnerable adults frequently, intensively and/or overnight (e.g. teaching, training, health care, supervision, advice, treatment and transportation)
- Any activity allowing contact with children or vulnerable adults that is in a *specified place*, frequently or intensively (e.g. school, care homes)
- Fostering and childminding
- Any activity in *defined areas of responsibility* (such as school governor, director of children's services, director of adult social services, trustees of certain charities)
- Regulated activity is when the activity is *frequent* (once a month or more), *intensive* (takes place on 3 or more days in a 30-day period), or *overnight*
- A barred individual *must not* undertake regulated activity

Controlled Activity:
- Ancillary support workers in *further education*, *NHS* and *adult social care* (e.g. domestic, caretaker, catering staff, receptionist) with frequent or intensive contact with children or vulnerable adults
- Those working for *specified organisations* with frequent access to sensitive records about children or vulnerable adults
- Barred people can be employed in controlled activity providing safeguards are in place

Key dates in implementing VBS

The following key dates were planned to be implemented from July 2010 – though implementation was suspended pending a review of the scheme on 15 June 2010. At the time of writing, the amended implementation timescale is not known.

12 October 2009:
- Current Government lists (PoCA, PoVA and List 99) will be replaced by two new ISA lists, one to cover working with children and one to cover working with vulnerable adults.
- Eligibility for enhanced CRB checks will expand for regulated positions.
- Standard CRB checks will no longer be available for those working or volunteering with children or vulnerable adults in regulated activity.
- Employers, social services and professional regulators will have a duty to notify ISA of all relevant information about individuals who may pose a threat to vulnerable groups.

From July 2010:
- Individuals seeking employment in regulated activity will need to register with the scheme. There will be a 5-year roll-out for existing staff. When they are registered they will be continually monitored and their status reassessed against new information.

- A new ISA/CRB application form will be issued.
- Employers will be required to ensure an individual in regulated activity is ISA registered *BEFORE* they take up appointment.
- Employers will be able to check an individual's ISA status online free of charge. They can also express an interest in a person's ISA registration status and will be notified should their status change whilst they are in their employment.
- It will become a crime for a barred individual to seek or undertake work with vulnerable groups, and for employers to knowingly take them on.

From November 2010:

- It will be a legal requirement for individuals to register with ISA if they work or volunteer with children or vulnerable adults.
- It will be a criminal offence for an employer to knowingly appoint or continue to employ anyone in regulated activity who is barred.
- It will also be a criminal offence for anyone to seek work in regulated activity with children or vulnerable adults if they are barred.

How will the ISA registration process work?

The ISA registration process and the VBS will have implications for all health care professionals. As a general guide anyone working in a caring role with a person with a learning disability will require a valid ISA registration and an enhanced CRB check as this will be considered 'regulated activity'.

If you are an employee or a volunteer who wants to work with vulnerable people, you need to apply for ISA registration. The ISA registration will be completed at the same time as the CRB Disclosure using the same form. The CRB gather all relevant information on each person. If no information is found, the CRB will issue ISA registration. If information is found, it is passed to the ISA for consideration.

ISA experts assess the information provided by the CRB and decide whether to give the individual ISA registration or put them on a barred list. ISA will also inform professional/regulatory bodies if someone is barred so that their professional registration can also be reviewed.

Continuous monitoring will ensure that if new information on an individual comes to light, the ISA will assess it and, if necessary, change their status. They will also advise the employer about that information. This will remove the need for repeating CRB checks for individual who remain in the same role as often happens now.

New staff will have their ISA registration processed as part of their pre-employment checks, unless they have already completed the ISA registration with a previous employer, in which case they will only need a new CRB.

COST

ISA registration will cost £64.00 – this will include the cost of lifetime ISA registration (£28.00) and the CRB check. The ISA registration is a one-off fee – future costs will only include the cost of the CRB currently £31.00 for standard and £36.00 for enhanced. Organisations will need to agree if they will fund this for all staff and some organisations may choose to make employees pay for some or all of this cost themselves.

**Please Note: At the time of writing a decision has still not been made as to whether individuals working in 'controlled activities' will be eligible for an Enhanced CRB Check. These positions are currently covered by a Standard Check.

If you have any queries about the Vetting and Barring Scheme you can contact: Tel: 0300 123 1111 or Email: scheme.info@homeoffice.gsi.gov.uk or check the following website for further guidance as issued: www.isa-gov.org.uk.

VALUES AND BELIEFS

Values

We explored in Chapter 1 how our values and beliefs influence our perception of people with a learning disability, and how this in turn influences the care we provide. Michael (2008) explained that 'The health and strength of a society can be measured by how well it cares for its most vulnerable members'. Michael continued to explain that:

'Health service staff, particularly those working in general healthcare, have very limited knowledge about learning disability. They are unfamiliar with the legislative framework, and commonly fail to understand that a right to equal treatment does not mean treatment should be the same. The health needs, communication problems, and cognitive impairment characteristic of learning disability in particular are poorly understood. Staff are not familiar with what help they should provide or from whom to get expert advice'.

BMA (2007, p. 27) reports that poor attitude and communication skills often have a negative impact on the experiences of disabled users. They highlight that the example set by senior staff is of great importance in enabling cultural change to be permanent within an organisation. Communication barriers may be the result of poor planning or a lack of resources and are not always in the control of an individual health care worker.

BMA (2007) explain that poor attitudes among workers within the health sector can contribute significantly to disabled people feeling isolated, disempowered and disengaged. This may be due to health care professionals:

- Not acknowledging the existence of disabling barriers
- Not realising that in order to achieve equal outcomes it is necessary to treat people differently by making adjustments
- Making assumptions about someone's wishes or what they think is in the best interests or about their capacity to make decisions
- Not listening to the person or seeing beyond the impairment
- Patronising the person because of their impairment
- Speaking directly to the person's carer or interpreter rather than the person themselves

They suggest that 'Patient care is more effective when a more holistic approach is adopted which enables a healthcare professional to look beyond a person's impairment and therefore open up communication by working in partnership with the patient'.

Normalisation

Normalisation is not about making people 'normal' – it is about enabling them to live normal valued lives. Wolf Wolfensberger (1972) is widely cited as the person who defined the principle of normalisation. He identified the core themes that devalued people with disability and suggested that 'handicapped people are socially devalued along with the elderly and sick'.

The work of Wolfensberger and his ideas on the devaluing of individuals led to the 'five principles of normalisation' developed by O'Brien (1987). These five principles are:

1. *Choice*: The experience of autonomy in making choices about small and large matter is part of all our daily lives. The choices we make are often based on the values and beliefs we have developed over our life time and define the person we are. Helping people with a learning disability to make 'real' choices about the decisions in their lives can be challenging and has been described by some carers as being a meaningless exercise.

   Kelly (2000) describes the example of encouraging a service user to choose the colour of the carpet in her bedroom. Samples were shown to the service users whose preferences were indicated by interpreting their eye gaze, pointing or verbal behaviour. However, if the service user does not have the understanding of what is being asked of them, then the choice is meaningless.

   (Helping people with a learning disability to make choices in a meaningful way is discussed in more detail in Chapter 3.)
2. *Respect*: Having a valued place in our community is an essential element in the promotion of our self-esteem. It is essential for those providing care and support to people with a learning disability that they ensure that information about what is happening in the world around them is explained in a way that they are able to understand and be given responsibility for managing the aspects of there life of which they are able. By affording respect and dignity to the person with a learning disability you promote an essential positive image of the person to the general public.
3. *Community presence*: The experience of living an ordinary life using the same facilities and resources accessed by everyone else is an important aspect of normalisation principles.
4. *Personal competence*: For people with learning disabilities this means being able to develop and enhance skills that promote independence and acceptance by others.
5. *Relationships*: Having a network of friendships and acquaintances is generally a highly valued aspect of community living for most of us. Having contact with our immediate family is also very important as is having a social life and, for some people, socialising independently.

For many people with learning disabilities their access to relationships and socialising outside their immediate environment can be minimal. It is not only the opportunity to develop relationships and access community facilities to meet new people that is challenging but having the appropriate support to help the individual develop the skills necessary to make and maintain relationships. It is for those supporting people with a learning disability to acknowledge the need for relationships and access to appropriate social networks.

These five principles provide the framework by which service provision for people with learning disabilities has been based in the years since they were developed.

Unfortunately the term 'normalisation' has become confused with the aim to 'make people normal' or to enforce behaviours that 'normal people do'. The misconception about the principles behind normalisation theory have led to some people with learning disabilities finding themselves not having their needs met because they are unable to comply with services that do not acknowledge that they need to be adapted to meet their needs. Normalisation does not mean changing the individual to become 'normal' but adapting the environment to meet the needs of the person with a learning disability within ordinary services.

One of the dilemmas that often arises is the issue of age appropriateness: When is it OK to display a soft toy on the bed or listen to/sing nursery rhymes to pass the time in the waiting room?

Nind and Hewitt (1994) explore the concept that age appropriateness is about behaviour that is culturally normal for an adult and how can we define this. How many adults have soft toys that they display happily in their own homes or enjoy a light-hearted playful game with their partner? It seems that it is about the decisions we make as to what we believe is behaviour that is OK to display privately or in public. Therefore when we are considering issues for the person we are supporting with regard to enabling the person in a respectful way we must ensure that whatever strategy we adopt does not devalue the person in anyway to the onlooker.

Reflective Learning Point:

Nind and Hewitt ask the question:

'Does doing this devalue the person in the eyes of the onlooker, and what should be our attitude toward that possibility?'

Our drive should not be to make the person 'normal', but to respect the persons preferred choices and to support the onlooker in their understanding of the person as they are and encourage the onlooker to value those choices. However, it is important to ensure that by respecting the individual in this way we do not endorse the stereotype of the person with a learning disability being a perpetual child.

Ethical and Political Case Study 6 – Normalisation 1

Gary is 32 years old and has profound learning disabilities and autism. He is waiting in the outpatients department for his consultation. Gary suffers from acute anxiety when he is in unfamiliar situations. When he is anxious he screams loudly and bangs his head on the floor. When he is anxious Gary sits on the floor rocking and likes to quietly sing nursery rhymes to himself.

When his carer notices that Gary is starting to become anxious she quietly takes Gary to a quiet area in the waiting room and sings his favourite song. Gary finds this reassuring and is able to sit until it is his turn to be seen.

This example may on first impression be considered inappropriate in a public area. However, if you consider what is the likely outcome of leaving Gary to console himself, that being Gary may start to scream or rock himself on the floor, this is more likely to draw unfavourable attention to Gary than his carer gently singing to him.

Ethical and Political Case Study 7 – Normalisation 2

Jenny has newly diagnosed diabetes and COPD and is in hospital because she has developed a severe chest infection. At home she has a reward chart that the care staff award her when she is compliant with her blood testing. She keeps the charts on her wall in her bedroom. In hospital Jenny has been refusing to have her blood taken and her carer suggests the use of sticker charts.

It is important in this case to recognise the difference between the sensitive display of Jenny's charts in her bedroom to the public display if the charts were to be placed on the wall near her bed on the ward. In this case it would be more appropriate that the stickers are in a book so that her care staff can view them when she visits and she can show them to health care staff but they are not visible to other patients who may view this and Jenny in a childlike way.

Therefore when considering the principles of normalisation in health care it is important to remember that people with learning disabilities should not by virtue of their disability be deprived of their right to health care. Health care professionals need to become aware of how they provide their service and acknowledge that there may be times when the way that service is provided may need to be adapted to meet the needs of an individual.

POLITICAL ISSUES AFFECTING SERVICE PROVISION IN BOTH LEARNING DISABILITY AND SECONDARY CARE SERVICES

This section explores how national policy has influenced the way that services are provided to people with a learning disability and a number of the key polices are highlighted.

As outlined in Chapter 1, historically some people with learning disabilities have been previously cared for in institutional settings. Not only was the institution their home, but all their social and health needs were catered for within the institution, with those individuals having little if indeed any contact with community health or social services. The doctor visited the wards, people were admitted to the institution hospital ward for treatment, and women had their babies all without leaving the locality of the institution.

The training of nurses for people with a learning disability in this setting was primarily based on a medical model of care with an emphasis on the assessment, planning, implementation and evaluation of health care. All learning disability nurses trained specifically to focus on the holistic assessment of people with learning disabilities.

In the 1960s, there were 65,000 people with a learning disability living in long-stay hospitals (Department of Health 2007a, p. 13). Since the policy of de-institutionalisation introduced in the 1970s led to closure of the long-stay hospitals, the service for people with learning disabilities has undergone numerous changes in its provision. Department of Health (2007a, p. 13) highlights this has resulted in 'dramatic changes in the lifestyle, experiences, expectations and aspirations of people with learning disabilities'. Learning disability nursing teams, specifically focused on providing health care for people with learning disabilities, have responded to these changes by developing a variety of services in community settings.

The significant change in the provision of services from long-stay hospitals to specialist community heath and social care provision, and to the current commissioning strategy of an increase in the purchasing of services from the independent sector, has impacted on the level of specialist general health assessment from skilled learning disability professionals. There is also an ongoing consideration as to whether the care provided for a person with a learning disability relates to health or social care needs. In practice, the majority of people with a learning disability have both these needs and need support from both specialist health and social care professionals to meet their needs.

There is growing evidence suggesting that people with learning disabilities have health needs that cannot be met by their social carers alone. This is possibly due to the inexperience of those supporting people with learning disabilities who may not have the skills to identify ill-health, or not having the skills to manage the patient in health care situations. There is also evidence to suggest that the health needs of these individuals are multiple, complex and difficult to establish without the depth of understanding of a skilled professional.

The needs of people with a learning disability often extend well beyond any 'intervention or procedure'. Those with complex needs require a service provided by professionals specifically trained to understand their biological, psychological and social needs. The need for regular health checks for people with a learning disability was highlighted in the 2006 White Paper 'Our Health, Our Care, Our Say' (Department of Health 2006).

The BMA (2007) report on 'Disability equality within healthcare' outlined the role of health care professionals in ensuring that the NHS is free from discrimination. They stated that (p. viii) 'the NHS should aim to provide equitable access to healthcare and work towards ensuring equality of health outcome for all patients' and outlined a number of ways that health care professionals can meet the needs of disabled people in health care.

For 2008/09 NHS Employers and the General Practitioner Committee of the BMA agreed five new clinical directed enhanced services (DES) as part of contract negotiations (NHS Employers and BMA 2009). The DES focus on the health and service priorities of the Department of Health that will benefit patients and includes a DES for people with a learning disability. The DES encourages GP practices to identify those people within their practice who have a moderate to severe learning disability and to offer them an annual health check.

GPs will be paid a bonus of £100 per health check completed. A similar scheme was already operating in Wales, which had helped to identify a host of previously undiagnosed conditions such as diabetes, asthma and high blood pressure. Though Mencap commented that GPs should be doing these health checks as part of their standard contract the BMA reported that 'these check ups are over and above the normal work'.

BBC news: 04.11.2008 – http://news.bbc.co.uk/1/hi/health/7707769.stm.

Whilst the political case can be argued to question why health services should be paid additional funds through a Directed Enhanced Service (or Local Enhanced Service) to provide health care to people with a learning disability that they are entitled to receive anyway, the evidence demonstrates that this does improve access to health care and therefore improves the health and well-being of people with a learning disability.

The changes in service provision for people with learning disabilities make it essential as highlighted by Sir Jonathon Michael (2008) and the Health Service Ombudsman report (2009) that 'all health services work in partnership with learning disability nurses to ensure that the services are appropriate and responsive to the needs of people with learning disabilities'.

Current policy recognises that there are problems for people with learning disabilities accessing mainstream services and that these services need to be equipped with the skills required to meet their needs.

Key policy documents

There have been a number of relevant policy and good practice guidance documents specifically aimed at health care professionals to highlight the issues affecting people with learning disabilities and their experience when accessing primary and secondary health services. The following are some of the key publications:

- Department of Health (2001) *Valuing People: A New Strategy for Learning Disability for the 21st Century*
- Mencap (2004) *Treat Me Right*
- Disability Rights Commission (2006) *Equal Treatment: Closing the Gap*
- Mencap (2007) *Death by Indifference*
- Sir Jonathan Michael MB, BS, FRCP, FKC (2008) *Healthcare for All*
- Health Service Ombudsman (2009) *Six Lives: The Provision of Public Services to People with Learning Disabilities*

Each of these key policies will be summarised in this section with the important issues highlighted.

Valuing people

The national learning disability White Paper, *Valuing People: A New Strategy for Learning Disability for the 21st Century*, outlined an overall aim for health for people with learning disabilities which is:

> **To enable people with a learning disability to access a health service designed around their individual needs, with fast convenient care delivered to a consistently high standard, and with additional support where necessary.**
>
> (Department of Health 2001)

The strategy sets out the Government's proposals for improving the lives of people with learning disabilities and their families and carers, based on the four basic tenets of 'recognition of their *rights* as citizens, social *inclusion* in local communities, *choice* in their daily lives and real opportunities to be *independent*'.

Valuing People outlines the requirements of councils and Primary Care Trusts in providing services to meet the needs of people with a learning disability. Objectives outlined in 'Valuing People' that are of particular relevance to the provision of health care include:

- 2.2: All public services will treat people with learning disabilities as individuals with respect for their dignity and challenge discrimination on all grounds including disability.
- 4.4: Making sure that all agencies work in partnership with carers, recognising that carers themselves have needs that must be met.
- 5.2: Enabling mainstream NHS services, with support from specialist learning disability staff, to meet the general and specific health needs of people with learning disabilities.
- 5.16: Carers should be treated as full partners by all agencies involved.

Key Health Objectives outlined in Chapter 6 (p. 59) include:

- Equal access to mainstream health services.
- Access to health services designed to meet individual needs with additional support where necessary.
- Ensuring all people with a learning disability are registered with a GP and that they have a health action plan including details of the need for health interventions: oral/dental health, mobility, vision, hearing, nutrition and emotional needs as well as details of medication taken and records of any screening tests.
- The appointment of health facilitators to support people with learning disabilities in getting the health care they need.
- Ensuring clear guidance on consent issues is available and accessible.
- National service frameworks applying equally to people with learning disabilities to ensure that they benefit from these initiatives.

Treat me right

The Mencap (2004) report 'Treat Me Right!' exposed the unequal health care that people with a learning disability often received from health care professionals. It put the case for better health care for people with a learning disability and argued that despite the fact that many policy reports and recommendations had been made to improve the situation little had actually changed. The report summarised what is known about the health needs of people with a learning disability and described numerous examples of people with a learning disability accessing health services.

Mencap highlighted negative experiences and made recommendations about what needed to be done to make sure that people with a learning disability get the treatment they need. They highlighted the issue of 'diagnostic overshadowing' when 'doctors wrongly believe that a presenting problem is as a result of the learning disability and that not much can be done about it'. They also found a lack of understanding and training among hospital staff. The report concluded that urgent action was needed to improve the health of people with a learning disability and address the problem of health inequalities. They also called for an inquiry into the premature deaths of people with a learning disability.

Equal treatment – closing the gap

Despite the previous policy drivers, the Disability Rights Commission (DRC 2006) investigation into health care given to people with mental health problems and learning disabilities showed that they often get worse treatment than others. The investigation examined 8 million health records and showed that people with learning disabilities and mental health problems are more likely to have a major illness, to develop a serious health condition younger and to die sooner than the rest of the population. Such people were less likely to have routine tests and screening to pick up signs of a problem in its early stages and fewer health investigations. They were also likely to face real barriers when accessing services. (http://news.bbc.co.uk/1/hi/health/5335722.stm.)

Death by indifference

This Mencap (2007) report was produced as a follow-up to 'Treat Me Right'. The report set out what it believed was 'institutional discrimination' within the NHS and that 'people with a learning disability get worse health care than non-disabled people'. The report outlined six case studies of people with a learning disability who had died whilst in hospital and raised serious concerns about the way people with a learning disability were treated within the health care system.

The report explained that despite evidence of health inequalities and documentation of early deaths nothing had been done and no action had been taken to address the issues – that is why the report was called Death by indifference – and called for an independent investigation into the deaths.

Reflective Learning Point:

Obtain a copy of 'Death by indifference' and read the accounts of the six people who died. Consider if this could happen in your area of work and what could be done to prevent this happening.

Health care for all

The complaints made by Mencap lead to the setting up of the independent inquiry into access to health care for people with learning disabilities led by Sir Jonathan Michael, MB, BS, FRCP (London) FKC, commissioned by the then Secretary of State for Health Patricia Hewitt. Sir Michael's report 'Healthcare for All' was published in July 2008.

The inquiry found 'convincing evidence that people with learning disabilities have higher levels of unmet need and receive less effective treatment, despite the fact that the Disability Discrimination Act and Mental Capacity Act set out a clear legal framework for the delivery of equal treatment'. Witnesses described examples of discrimination, abuse and neglect across the range of health services.

This report highlighted that 'What matters is that people with learning disabilities are included as equal citizens, with equal rights of access to equally effective treatment'. Whilst the six cases highlighted by Mencap were seen as shocking there was also evidence of good practice and what was needed was to ensure that this good practice was encouraged to spread more widely.

The report makes 10 principal recommendations. The aim of these recommendations is to achieve an effective, fair system of general health care for people with learning disabilities.

All 10 recommendations are summarised in Chapter 1 and the following are highlighted as the key considerations for general hospital health care providers:

Recommendation 2 – All health care organisations including the Department of Health should ensure they collect the data and information necessary to allow people with a learning disability to be identified by the health service and their pathways of care tracked.

Recommendation 3 – Family and other carers should be involved as a matter of course in the provision of treatment and care, unless a good reason is given, and Trust Boards should ensure that reasonable adjustments are made to enable and support carers to do this effectively.

Recommendation 7 – Inspectors and regulators of the health service should develop and extend their monitoring of the standard of general health services provided for people with learning disabilities, in both the hospital sector and the community where primary care providers are located. The aim is to support appropriate, reasonable adjustments to general health services for adults and children with learning disabilities and their families and to ensure compliance with, and enforcement of, all aspects of the Disability Discrimination Act.

Recommendation 9 – Section 242 of the National Health Service Act 2006 requires NHS bodies to involve and consult patients and the public in the planning and development of services, and in decisions affecting the operation of services. All Trust Boards should ensure that the views and interests of people with learning disabilities and their carers are included.

Recommendation 10 – All Trust Boards should demonstrate that they have systems in place to deliver effective, 'reasonably adjusted' health services. This should include arrangements to provide advocacy for all those who need it, and to secure effective representation on PALS from all client groups including people with learning disabilities.

Acute hospitals can respond to these recommendations by implementing the good practice examples described in Sir Michael's report those being:

- The development of policy for supporting people with learning disabilities in the acute hospital.
- The development of patient profiles or communication passports inform health care staff of the patients needs if they are unable to communicate their needs themselves.
- Promotion of acute liaison nurses to support people with learning disabilities and to advise acute services.
- Risk alert cards in case files or flagging systems on computerised systems that indicate the person has a learning disability.

Reflective Learning Point:

How many of these recommendations would you be confident could be applied to your area of work/hospital at the present time?

Six lives

In March 2009, the Ombudsman published 'Six Lives: The Provision of Public Services to People With Learning Disabilities'. This shocking report gave an overview and summary of the investigation reports of the six cases highlighted in Mencap's report 'Death by Indifference' published in 2007.

The Ombudsman's report illustrates some significant and distressing failures in service provision across both health and social care services which is believed to have led to situations where people with learning disabilities have experienced prolonged suffering and inappropriate care. Hospitals were criticised for the inadequate care and treatment given to people with learning disabilities as well as the way they looked into complaints.

The report shows the impact of organisational behaviour when:

- Services do not make the reasonable adjustments to the provision of care to meet individuals needs
- Failure to understand the law in relation to disability discrimination and human rights
- There is a lack of leadership, 'to maintain a focus on the experience of and outcomes for people with learning disabilities' (p. 9).

The areas of concern included:

- Communication
- Partnership working and coordination
- Relationships with family and carers
- Failure to follow routine procedures
- Quality management
- Advocacy

The Ombudsman said that there was sufficient policy and guidance available, but agencies were not following it and, as a result, were in breach of human rights and disability discrimination laws. The report recommends that all NHS and social care organisations in England should review urgently:

1. The effectiveness of the systems they have in place to enable them to understand and plan to meet the full range of needs of people with learning disabilities in their areas.
2. The capacity and capability of the services they provide and/or commission for their local populations to meet the additional and often complex needs of people with learning disabilities.

Reflective Learning Point:

'No one took a proactive approach to owning and resolving problems by making reasonable adjustments and seeking urgent solutions' (p. 25).

The Ombudsman's report also raises the issue of the shortcomings in the lack of understanding of the legislation and guidance available to health care professions when providing care to people with learning disabilities. This may be due to the way that this information is disseminated to staff and also the relevance that staff pay to informing themselves about the information and acting upon it.

Reflective Learning Point:

Get a copy of the Ombudsman's report and consider the areas that apply to your practice as a health care professional.

Leadership

It is essential that senior health care managers and medical professionals make efforts to address health care access (BMA 2007). This can be achieved by having diversity or specific disability champions whose role it is to ensure that all health care professional and service providers have access to appropriate advice, support and training and act as an advocate within their organisation to advocate for people with disabilities.

This should not be a replacement for inclusive policy and procedures, or individual professionals' responsibility to the patient, but should help to provide the safeguards essential to ensuring that the needs of people who are vulnerable for any reason are addressed, and appropriate adjustments made for their care.

INTERDISCIPLINARY APPROACHES AND PARTNERSHIP WORKING

Caring for people with a learning disability involves an inter-disciplinary approach with a number of health and social care professionals contributing a range of different skills. This section explores some of the key roles and outlines the different areas of expertise of some of the professionals involved.

The learning disability nurse and the health facilitation role

Learning disability nursing is one of four branches of nursing with pre-registration training courses over 3 years leading to a registered nurse qualification at either degree or diploma level. Community learning disability nurses have usually undertaken a BSc Community Specialist Practitioner course in addition to their registered nurse training. Many learning disability nurses also complete a range of advanced post-registration training courses in areas such as epilepsy, behavioural approaches, or psychosocial interventions. Learning disability nurses are the only professional group who are trained solely to address the needs of this vulnerable group and only around 25,000 nurses are registered in the UK to practice in learning disability specialism.

The Department of Health (2007a) defined learning disability nursing as 'a person-centred profession with the primary aim of supporting the well-being and social inclusion of people with learning disabilities through improving or maintaining physical and mental health'. They continue to explain that learning disability nurses 'act as champions for people with learning disabilities and their families. They undertake a range of activities to promote better health for people with learning disabilities. They do this by advising, teaching and supporting people with learning disabilities, their families and other professionals to enable people to live full and rewarding lives within their communities. They specifically provide nursing input and direct support to people with complex needs related to their learning disability. They work in a wide range of settings and work in partnership with people with learning disabilities and their families, as well as with other professionals, organisations and the wider community'.

Three main practice areas were identified for learning disability nurses:

- Health facilitation – supporting access to mainstream services
- Inpatient services – for example, assessment and treatment and secure services
- Specialist roles – in community teams

The range of activities undertaken includes health assessment, health promotion, advocacy, skills teaching, training other professionals, supporting families and carers, promoting disability awareness and equality, and contributing to the development of new services. As with other branches of nursing, modern matron, nurse prescriber and consultant nurse roles have all been established.

The UK Learning Disability Consultant Nurse Network (2006) states that 'learning disability nurses provide a crucial role in providing assessment, treatment, intervention, education and support for people with learning disabilities, their carers, general health services and others'.

Learning disability nursing is a values-based profession and Department of Health (2007a, p. 18) outlines the following specific person-centred values:

- The person with a learning disability must be at the centre of their care and be fully involved in all aspects of planning care and treatment
- Choice and self-determination must be supported by offering timely and appropriate information
- Recognising the contribution of family carers and providing support to them in their role is critical
- Working with those who provide paid support directly is key to ensuring that the health needs of people with learning disabilities are understood and healthy lifestyles are promoted
- People with learning disabilities have interrelated social, psychological, physical and spiritual needs
- Inequality in all aspects of the life of people with learning disabilities must be actively challenged
- Care must be provided in a way that is based on the best evidence available
- Health interventions should be provided in the person's everyday environment in the first instance and, where this is not possible, then within the least restrictive setting and as close to home as possible

They also outline a set of 15 benchmarks that demonstrate good practice in learning disability nursing which includes a need to 'support the provision of excellent physical and mental health care to people with learning disabilities in all settings'.

The ability to anticipate, interpret and change behaviour is a central component of learning disability nursing practice. These skills and competencies need to be considered in the context of factors such as determining capacity to consent, obtaining consent where appropriate and interpreting issues around distress.

One of the key aspects of the learning disability nurse role is to act as a 'Health Facilitator' for people with a learning disability. This role was first outlined in Valuing People (2001), which emphasised the need for specialist learning disability workers to take on a greater role in supporting people with learning disabilities to access mainstream health and other services. This role includes developing closer working relationships with primary and acute hospital service providers to achieve the overall aim of Valuing People. Community learning disability nurses in some areas are currently assisting GP practices in the development of learning disability registers with their practices and implementing annual health checks for people with learning disabilities. It is therefore essential that primary care services engage with learning disability nurses to ensure that they fully utilise the health check and ensure that identified needs are addressed.

Many learning disability nurses have developed expertise in additional areas, for example behavioural approaches, sexual health, counselling and psychotherapy, palliative care, complementary therapies and education. Therefore learning disability nurses are available to play a key role in translating the theoretical knowledge into practice and work in partnership with other health care professionals.

Department of Health (2007a, p. 31) highlighted an example of where two learning disability nurses were employed in the commissioning team of a Primary Care Trust working across the health community and with the local authority in developing and implementing the local joint strategic and commissioning plan. Their knowledge of learning disability was used to create a service specification, model of care and outcome measures to meet the health and social care needs whilst also ensuring quality of care and value for money.

Other examples outlined learning disability nurses working in (p. 37) independent sector settings undertaking quality and service development roles, and (p. 38) in formal care management roles meeting health related needs in local authority services.

Particular skills of learning disability nurses that are of relevance to health care professionals in primary care and acute settings are:

- Knowledge of a range of learning disability conditions and associated health conditions such as epilepsy
- Knowledge and understanding of the specific health needs of people with a learning disability
- Support to explain how and why people with a learning disability might be treated for health problems
- Understanding of what the disability means for the individual – enabling person-centred approaches to health care
- Consent to treatment and best interest decision making
- Anti-discriminatory practice and fair treatment
- Understanding and responding to challenging behaviour
- Training and education in disability issues
- Improving and supporting access to health care, including overcoming barriers to care
- Enhanced communication skills, and the development of accessible information tools

It is concerning to many learning disability nurses that nurse education is set to change radically to respond to the modernising of nursing careers agenda. In 2007, the Department of Health (2007b) announced plans for a framework for post-registration training for nurses that will align nursing careers with the National NHS careers framework and develop new career paths for nurses.

The case for change notes that health inequalities persist despite the efforts made to reduce the gap for vulnerable people such as people with learning disabilities. It is thought that learning disability nursing will be a specialist dimension of the long-term conditions pathway or psychosocial care. However, considering the concerns that the needs of people with learning disabilities are complex and difficult to establish, there is the possibility that the skills and knowledge attained through a 3-year dedicated pathway may be diminished in this new proposed programme, which could potentially lead to fragmentation of care to this vulnerable group.

Acute liaison nurse

The development of the acute liaison nurse role (as supported by Sir Jonathon Michael and the Healthcare Ombudsman) has been developing in some districts over the last 10 years. The acute liaison nurse is usually an experienced member of the community learning disability team with specific responsibility for service users accessing acute hospital services. For the majority of these posts this will be in addition to their community nursing duties, but for others their post will be dedicated to this role and some are even based within acute hospital trusts.

The scope of the role will be dependent on the location but the following are generally the key issues for acute liaison nurses.

- Support and advice for people with a learning disability accessing general hospital services
- Support relatives/family members/carers who are affected by the patient's illness/hospital stay
- Support and advice for the acute care staff in relation to personalised care and service delivery
- Promote collaboration between the agencies involved in service delivery to ensure effective seamless care
- Coordination of care at points of attendance, admission and discharge
- Education within clinical areas and contributing to programmes of education
- Enhance and develop standards of care for all patients with a learning disability attending the acute hospital
- Promotion of effective communication with those involved in the patient's care whether they are community- or hospital-based

The overall emphasis for the majority of acute liaison nurses is to influence the provision of services in general hospitals to ensure that the needs of people with learning disabilities are considered in all aspects of care delivery.

Pointu et al. (2009) see the role of the acute liaison nurses as 'championing the needs of this often invisible population by ensuring that care is effective, safe and compassionately tailored to meet the individual's needs'. The study by Pointu et al also identified that the acute liaison nurse contributes to a reduction of the length of stay in hospital and improvements in safety.

The provision of learning disability nursing differs within health care districts. Some nurses are based within integrated health and social work team; some will be linked to the Primary Care Trust. All Social Service departments and Primary Care Trusts will be able to identify the location of the learning disability nursing team in your area.

The value of this role was highlighted in 2008 by Elizabeth Edwards, a nurse (RGN), who wrote about her experiences of accessing hospital care with her severely disabled daughter. It was her opinion that 'every general hospital should have a learning disability liaison nurse on its staff to offer help and advice to the staff and relatives of patients with learning disabilities' (Edwards 2008).

Her daughter Ruth had Walker Warburg syndrome (WWS), which means she had complex needs, profound learning disabilities, epilepsy, visual and hearing problems. However, she explained that in spite of all her problems Ruth 'was a loving cheerful girl who made an impression on all who met her'.

Ruth died at the age of 24 and during the last 3 years of her life she had several hospital admissions. Edwards described this as 'All her hospital admissions seemed to be a battle for the nursing and medical staff to see her as a person'. Whilst there were examples of excellent care this was seen as the exception and in general the care she received was described as 'very poor' by Edwards, who felt she had to keep a close eye on her when she was in hospital. She described 'how much she would have appreciated it if the hospital had employed a learning disability nurse as a liaison nurse. Someone I could have spoken to and who would have understood Ruth's needs'.

This story highlights the importance of this role, not just for the individual but also for their family and carers, and for the support and advice that can be provided to other health care professionals.

Reflective Learning Point:

Can you think of a situation you may have experienced when caring for a person with a learning disability and how a learning disability nurse/acute liaison nurse could have helped with this?

Other professionals who can help

Working with people with a learning disability is a complex and multi-faceted task requiring a range of professionals with complementary skills working together to develop and provide quality services. We have summarised here the skills of some of the key professionals and the role they can contribute to the health care process.

Role of the speech and language therapist

Speech and language therapists (SALTs) work with a wide range of people who have communication and/or feeding difficulties including children with delayed/disordered communication, adults with acquired disorders, people with learning disabilities etc. Regardless of which client group they work with their role is to:

- Assess and diagnose communication and feeding/swallowing difficulties (communication difficulties can happen at any stage of the communication chain)
- Provide advice to client/carers/families and other professionals
- Carry out therapy in a range of different ways appropriate to client need, for example programmes, staff training, individual or group therapy

SALT may work with children in mainstream and specialist resources. Therapists working with adults support them in all appropriate settings, for example home, college, centre, work place etc.

A significant aspect of the role may be supporting carers to appreciate the level of language that a person can understand and use alternative/augmentative strategies when communicating. The role may also include providing training in these strategies, for example signing, objects of reference, using visuals and developing accessible information.

A SALT may be supporting people to express themselves by developing non-verbal and verbal communication and communication skills in areas such as social skill development, for example turn taking. A more familiar role for SALT, especially in acute hospital settings, is to assess and advise regarding feeding and swallowing difficulties. This can highlight some ethical and consent issues. They may advise changes to a person's diet, that is textures, consistencies, utensils etc.

Some people with a learning disability may have identified swallowing difficulties that have been managed in the community. For some individuals the risks of aspiration will be known and acknowledged with relevant risk assessment in place to support feeding with known swallowing difficulties. It is important to establish if this is the case if a person with a leaning disability is admitted, and if there are any concerns regarding swallowing.

It is strongly advisable to contact your local learning disability SALT to give advice on issues relating to people with learning disabilities who have swallowing difficulties. This was a key issue in the *Six Lives* report outlined earlier in the chapter.

SALT work as part of the multi-disciplinary team around specific clients or around particular issues, for example Mental Capacity Act, dementia assessment, care planning. They may carry out joint assessment with other professionals or provide advice/training as a team.

Consultant psychiatrist

A consultant psychiatrist usually works in a community mental health team which is involved in caring for people living in a certain geographical area. Team members include trainee psychiatrists, social workers, community psychiatric nurses, psychologists and others. Though most consultant psychiatrists work in the mental health field, some do specialise in working with people with a learning disability. Consultant psychiatrists specialise in dealing with people with mental health disorders and have expertise in assessing and treating a range of mental health problems. People with a learning disability have a high level of mental health issues in addition to their learning disability.

The consultant or the team will have patients referred to them by GPs and other professionals such as health visitors and social workers. Referrals are then allocated to various members in the team, depending on the nature of the individual's problems. The consultant has overall responsibility for the management of patients under the care of the team. The consultant will also often have responsibility for a certain number of patients in a hospital ward.

A consultant is approved under Section 12 of the Mental Health Act (1983), enabling them to recommend the involuntary detention of a patient who is severely ill in hospital in the interests of their health, their safety or the safety of others. Involuntary detention in hospital only occurs if two doctors and an approved social worker all agree that this is an appropriate thing to happen.

Clinical psychologists

Clinical psychologists deal with the psychological aspects of mental ill-health. They are involved in the assessment of the extent of impairment of brain function and in the rehabilitation following injury or trauma. They deal with brain injury, post-traumatic stress, memory problems and psychological disturbance.

They can test for most specific learning difficulties, including dyslexia, dyspraxia, attention-deficit/hyperactivity disorder, obsessive-compulsive disorder, autism and Asperger's syndrome. They also provide assessment and treatment for people with conditions such as depression and eating disorders.

Educational psychologists

Educational psychologists are concerned with children's learning and development, and with this focus they work mainly in schools, with teachers and parents. They carry out a range of tasks with the aim of enhancing children's learning. They offer psychological support and advice to enable teachers to help children more effectively and are aware of the range of social and curriculum factors which affect teaching and learning.

Psychotherapist

Psychotherapists are often linked to psychology or mental health services and provide specialist support to people in emotional and psychological distress. Some psychotherapists have a nursing background. Treatment and support is usually sessional and short term, using therapies such as cognitive-behavioural therapy and expressive art and play therapies.

Psychiatric nurses

Psychiatric nurses work with adults and children who have a variety of mental health problems. Usually they are based within a mental health team which may be hospital- or community-based. They work with people in their own home or in residential units or special hospitals and secure units. They provide assessment and care for people with acute mental distress or who have enduring mental illness.

Social care staff

Social care staff provide direct care and support to people with learning disabilities in a variety of settings, from the person's own home to residential care, day care and respite care. They may be paid by the person through a direct payment scheme or the care staff may be provided by social services. More social care staff today are provided from private care agencies and the voluntary sector. Social care staff will be trained to a varied level of competence. Some staff will have received little if any training specifically in caring for people with learning disabilities.

Social workers and care managers

Social workers and care managers are employed by social services and their role is to assess, commission and review packages of care to meet the needs of people with learning disabilities. The role of the social worker has radically changed over the last 5 years and few social workers now provide a traditional supportive role to people with learning disabilities. Some social workers will focus specifically on safeguarding vulnerable adult issues or will be Deprivation of Liberty assessors or Approved mental heath professionals involved in the assessment and support of people with learning disabilities and mental health needs.

Some people with a learning disability will have an appointed social worker but it is likely that if a person with a learning disability is admitted to hospital and has changes to the care they need on discharge that they will require a referral to social services.

WHERE DO WE GO FROM HERE?

As has been highlighted throughout this book, general hospitals are responsible for providing good quality health care services to meet the needs of people with a learning disability. They need to be flexible and responsive to individual needs and are also required (by law) to make reasonable adjustments to ensure that appropriate care is provided. We have also explored the current evidence base which shows that this does not always happen effectively and highlighted key actions that staff working in general hospitals can take to identify and meet health needs.

Novice to expert

We recognise that working with people with a learning disability is a learning process for people who do not have any specific disability training. The evidence base in Chapter 1 showed that more exposure and time spent with people with a learning disability leads to the development of a more positive attitude, the development of skills and competencies and increased confidence.

Benner (1984) outlines this process as developing 'from novice to expert' and applies a model of skill acquisition developed by Dreyfus in the development of nursing practice. Myrtle Aydelotte, in the foreword to Benner's book, explains that we 'learn what expert nurses do in specific patient care situations and how beginners and experts do it differently; we also learn how, as their clinical careers develop, nurses themselves change their intellectual orientation, integrate and sort out their knowledge, and refocus their decision-making on a different basis than the process-orientated one they were taught'. Whilst this book was written with a nursing reference the principles of learning and development of clinical practice are transferable to other health care professional groups.

The Dreyfus model of skill acquisition suggests that we pass through five levels of proficiency in acquiring and developing our skills:

Level 1 – Novice
Level 2 – Advanced beginner
Level 3 – Competent
Level 4 – Proficient
Level 5 – Expert

Reflective Learning Point:

What level would you describe yourself at with regard to your current knowledge and skill for working with a person with a learning disability?

Benner (p. 13) describes how these different levels reflect changes in three general aspects of skilled performance:

1. A movement from reliance on abstract principles to the use of past concrete experience as paradigms.
2. A change in the learner's perception of the demand situation, in which the situation is seen as less and less as a compilation of equally relevant bits, and more and more as a complete whole in which only certain parts are relevant.
3. A passage from *detached* observer to *involved* performer. The performer no longer stands outside the situation but is now engaged in the situation.

Reflective Learning Point:

Think of a situation that you may have encountered early in your health career:

- How did you react at the time?
- How would you react now?
- What makes the difference?

Much of this skilled performance is best developed through real-life experience rather than through formal learning, e.g. from lectures or books. Novices and advanced beginners need 'rules' to follow in the beginning but as they progress through the skill acquisition process more 'intuitive responses' develop. Preceptorship, or working with a more experienced person, can help the learning process.

Proficient and expert practitioners grasp and understand situations as a whole and develop a perception (learned and based on their experience) of what is the right thing to do in a given situation. This holistic understanding enables the person to pick up on the important aspects of health care and know what to deal with first. The expert performer is highly proficient and has an intuitive grasp of each situation and often a 'gut feeling' of what is the right thing to do in any given situation. They 'just know' what to do though how they do this is not always easy to put into words and explain to someone else.

Whilst not everyone needs to be an expert, all health care professionals can develop the basic skills required to work effectively with a person with a learning disability. What initially appears confusing can be dealt with confidently with experience. The individual, their family/carer and learning disability professionals can offer the support and advice needed.

We have summarised the key competencies in a personal checklist below and also include an organisational checklist based on best practice in providing health care services to people with a learning disability (see Tables 6.1–6.3).

CONCLUSION

This chapter explored the key ethical and political aspects of caring for people with a learning disability and considered how these impact on the health care process and quality of care provided.

The issues of professional accountability and ethical decision making highlighted the personal and professional responsibilities of all health care professionals, and the implications for their practice. Special consideration is needed to ensure the safeguarding of children and vulnerable adults.

Exploration of the national policy framework highlighted how this has influenced and changed the provision of service to people with a learning disability over the past 40 years. Some quite shocking examples of poor care were highlighted with the Healthcare Ombudsman (2009) reporting on an investigation into the deaths of six people with a learning disability whilst in hospital care.

Approaches to partnership working and the range of other professional who can help were identified with brief information provided about individual roles. The chapter concludes with consideration of how health care professionals working in general hospitals can progress from 'Novice to Expert' in developing their skills and competencies and confidence in working with people with a learning disability. Personal and organisation checklists and a benchmark for good practice are provided for self-assessment.

Table 6.1 Health care professional personal best practice checklist

All health care professionals working with people with a learning disability should

Action	√	Date
Develop their knowledge and understanding of the specific health needs of people with a learning disability		
Attend disability awareness training sessions		
Spend time working with people with a learning disability to develop confidence and a more positive attitude		
Develop a range of communication skills and tools to enable them to overcome barriers to communication		
Ensure they are up-to-date and familiar with guidance about informed decision making and consent issues		
Develop an awareness of behavioural issues and ways of working with these		
Develop skills in assessing pain in people with a learning disability		
Develop an awareness of the principles of advocacy and empowerment and use these in their professional practice		
Have knowledge and contact details of local learning disability teams and other professionals who can help		
Contribute to a resource pack of information in your area of practice to support effective care for people with a learning disability		

Table 6.2 Organisations best practice checklist

Action	√	Date
Provide learning disability awareness training for staff		
Develop clear policies and guidance for staff that include core principles about how to work with people with a learning disability		
Identify people in the organisation with a lead responsibility for learning disability aspects of care		
Acute liaison nurse (learning disabilities) in post		
Agree a standard pre-admission assessment process for people with a learning disability and documentation to highlight additional needs at an early stage		
Develop local care pathways for services, especially for elective admissions, emergency admissions, outpatient attendance, theatre and recovery, and discharge planning		
Provide a person-centred approach to care planning with a focus on individual need		
Identify and address the needs of carers of people with a learning disability		
Produce accessible information about the hospital and health care procedures		
Provide clear guidance about how staff can make reasonable adjustments and also ensure compliance with disability equality legislation, supported by additional funding where required		
Monitor how many patients with a learning disability are admitted and record how well the admission and the additional support went – and use the information to inform future service provision		
Consult with people with a learning disability and their family/carers – Ask them how the service needs to be and involve them in planning and developing services		

Table 6.3 A2A essence of care benchmark

Factor		Benchmark of good practice
1	Information to access hospital	Good, clear up-to date information using a variety of methods is available at an appropriate time to support access
2	Specialist knowledge and skills	Access to specialist knowledge and skills will be available 24 hours a day
3	Attitudes and behaviours	All staff will treat individuals with respect all of the time
4	Support	Patients and carers receive the support required for that period of care
5	Information	Comprehensive up-to-date information accompanies the patient to allow for continuity and coordination of care
6	Communication	All practicable steps are taken to communicate effectively with patients and their carers
7	Awareness raising	All staff undertake training/development to raise their awareness of learning disabilities
8	Equipment	Patients/clients have access to the equipment need to meet their individual needs and are supported to use it
9	Balancing observation and privacy in a safe environment	Patients/clients are cared for in an environment that balances safe observation and privacy
10	Activity	Patients needs for activity are assessed and provided for on an individual basis

A2A.

Summary of Key Learning Points

The key learning points are:
- All health care professionals are accountable for providing a high quality of care to every person they work with
- The fact that a person has a learning disability does not mean they should be treated any differently than anyone else
- Health care decision making should be based on the basic ethical concepts of avoiding harm, respect for individual rights and acting always in the person's best interests
- There are five principles of normalisation which require health care professionals to adapt the environment in order to meet the needs of the person with a learning disability within ordinary services
- Leadership and the use of diversity or specific disability champions can help to develop person-centred services
- Learning disability nurses and a range of other professionals can offer good support and advice to general hospital staff
- The overall aim for health care professionals is **'To enable people with a learning disability to access a health service designed around their individual needs, with fast convenient care delivered to a consistently high standard, and with additional support where necessary'.**

(Valuing People 2001)

Links to KSF Competencies – Chapter 6

	Level descriptors			
Core dimensions	1	2	3	4
1 – Communication	Communicate with a limited range of people on day-to-day matters	Communicate with a range of people on a range of matters	Develop and maintain communication with people about difficult matters and/or in difficult situations	Develop and maintain communication with people on complex matters, issues and ideas and/or in complex situations
2 – Personal and people development	Contribute to own personal development	Develop own skills and knowledge and provide information to others to help their development	Develop oneself and contribute to the development of others	Develop oneself and others in areas of practice
3 – Health safety and security	Assist in maintaining own and others' health, safety and security	Monitor and maintain health, safety and security of self and others	Promote, monitor and maintain best practice in health, safety and security	Maintain and develop an environment and culture that improves health, safety and security
4 – Service improvement	Make changes in own practice and offer suggestions for improving services	Contribute to the improvement of services	Appraise, interpret and apply suggestions, Recommendations and directives to improve services	Work in partnership with others to develop, take forward and evaluate direction, policies and strategies
5 – Quality	Maintain the quality of own work	Maintain quality in own work and encourage others to do so	Contribute to improving quality	Develop a culture that improves quality
6 – Equality and diversity	Act in ways that support equality and value diversity	Support equality and value diversity	Promote equality and value diversity	Develop a culture that promotes equality and values diversity

	Level descriptors			
Health and well-being	1	2	3	4
HWB1 – Promotion of health and well-being and prevention of adverse effects on health and well-being	Contribute to promoting health and well-being and preventing adverse effects on health and well-being	Plan, develop and Implement approaches to promote health and well-being and prevent adverse effects on health and well-being	Plan, develop and implement programmes to promote health and well-being and prevent adverse effects on health and well-being	Promote health and well-being and prevent adverse effects on health and well-being through contributing to the development, implementation and evaluation of related policies

HWB2 – Assessment and care planning to meet health and well-being needs	Assist in the assessment of people's health and well-being needs	Contribute to assessing health and well-being needs and planning how to meet those needs	Assess health and well-being needs and develop, monitor and review care plans to meet specific needs	Assess complex health and well-being needs and develop, monitor and review care plans to meet those needs
HWB3 – Protection of health and well-being	Recognise and report situations where there might be a need for protection	Contribute to protecting people at risk	Implement aspects of a protection plan and review its effectiveness	Develop and lead on the implementation of an overall protection plan
HWB4 – Enablement to address health and well-being needs	Help people meet daily health and well-being needs	Enable people to meet ongoing health and well-being needs	Enable people to address specific needs in relation to health and well-being	Empower people to realise and maintain their potential in relation to health and well-being
HWB5 – Provision of care to meet health and well-being needs	Undertake care activities to meet individuals' health and well-being needs	Undertake care activities to meet the health and well-being needs of individuals with a greater degree of dependency	Plan, deliver and evaluate care to meet people's health and well-being needs	Plan, deliver and evaluate care to address people's complex health and well-being needs
HWB6 – Assessment and treatment planning	Undertake tasks related to the assessment of physiological and psychological functioning	Contribute to the assessment of physiological and psychological functioning	Assess physiological and psychological functioning and develop, monitor and review related treatment plans	Assess physiological and psychological functioning when there are complex and/or undifferentiated abnormalities, diseases and disorders and develop, monitor and review related treatment plans
HWB7 – Interventions and treatments	Assist in providing interventions and/or treatments	Contribute to planning, delivering and monitoring interventions and/or treatments	Plan, deliver and evaluate interventions and/or treatments	Plan, deliver and evaluate interventions and/or treatments when there are complex issues and/or serious illness

Department of Health (2004). Reproduced under the terms of the Click-Use Licence.

REFERENCES

A2A – Access to Acute: A network for staff working with people with learning disabilities to support access to acute medical treatment (2009). Available at http://www.nnldn.org.uk/a2a/ Contact: rick.robson@sssft.nhs.uk.

Benner P (1984) *From Novice to Expert*. Addison-Wesley Publishing Company, California.

BMA (2007) *Disability Equality in Healthcare*. BMA, London.

Chaloner C (2007) Ethics – it's everybody's business! *RCN Magazine*, Spring, p. 29.

Collis SP (2006) The importance of truth-telling in health care. *Nursing Standard*, 20(17), 41–54.

Council for Healthcare Regulatory Excellence (2009) *Clear Sexual Boundaries between Healthcare Professionals and Patients: Information for Patients and Carers*. NHS Employers, London.

Department for Constitutional Affairs (2005) *Mental Capacity Act 2005*. The Stationary Office, London.

Department of Health (1983) *Mental Health Act*. HMSO, London.

Department of Health (2001) *Valuing Peop*. Department of Health, London.

Department of Health (2004) *The NHS Knowledge and Skills Framework (NHS KSF) and the Development Review Process. Appendix 1: Overview of the NHS KSF*. HMSO, London.

Department of Health (2006) *Our Health, Our Care, Our Say*. Department of Health, London.

Department of Health (2007a) *Good Practice in Learning Disability Nursing*. Department of Health, London.

Department of Health (2007b) *Towards a Framework for Post-Registration Nursing Careers – Consultation Document*. The Stationery Office, London.

Department of Health (2009a) *The NHS Constitution*. Department of Health, London.

Department of Health (2009b) *The Statement of NHS Accountability* (for England). Department of Health, London.

Department of Health (Darzi report) (2008) *High Quality Care for All: NHS Next Step Review*. Department of Health, London.

Department of Health and the Home Office (2000) *No Secrets: Guidance on Developing and Implementing Multi-agency Policies and Procedures to Protect Vulnerable Adults from Abuse*. Department of Health, London.

Disability Rights Commission (2006) *Equal Treatment: Closing the Gap*. DRC, London.

Edwards E (2008) Dignity. *NMC News*, July, p. 8.

General Medical Council (2001) *Good Medical Practice*. GMC, London.

Gates B (2005) *Care Planning and Delivery in Intellectual Disability Nursing*. Blackwell Publishing, Oxford.

Healthcare Commission (2007a) *Investigation into Services for People with Learning Disabilities at Cornwall Partnership NHS Trust*. Healthcare Commission, London. Available at www.healthcarecommission.org.uk.

Healthcare Commission (2007b) *Investigation into the Service for People with Learning Disabilities Provided by Sutton and Merton Primary Care Trust*. Healthcare Commission, London. Available at www.healthcare commission.org.uk.

Jenkins R and Davis R (2004) The abuse of adults with learning disabilities and the role of the learning disability nurse. *Learning Disability Practice*, 7(2), 30–38.

Kelly A (2000) *Working with Adults with a Learning Disability*. Wilmslow Press, Oxon.

Mencap (2004) *Treat Me Right!* Mencap, London.

Mencap (2007) *Death by Indifference*. Mencap, London.

Michael J (2008) *Healthcare for All. Report of the Independent Inquiry into Access to Healthcare for People with Learning Disabilities*. HMSO, London.

NHS Employers (2008) *NHS Employment Check Standards*. NHSE, London.

NHS Employers and BMA (2009) *Clinical Directed Enhanced Services (DESs) for GMS Contract 2008/09. Guidance and Audit Requirements*. NHSE, London.

Nind M and Hewitt D (1994) *Access to Communication: Developing the Basics of Communication with People with Severe Learning Difficulties Through Intensive Interaction*. David Fulton Publishers, London.

Nursing and Midwifery Council (2002) *Practitioner-Client Relationships and the Prevention of Abuse*. NMC, London.

Nursing and Midwifery Council (2007) *Covert Administration of Medicines – Disguising Medicine in Food and Drink*. NMC, London.

O'Brien J (1987) A guide to life-style planning: using the activities catalogue to integrate services and natural support systems. In: Bellamy G and Wilcox B (eds) *A Comprehensive Guide to the Activities Catalogue: An Alternative Curriculum for Youth and Adults with Severe Disabilities*. Paul H. Brookes, Baltimore, pp. 175–189.

Parliamentary and Health Service Ombudsman (2009) *Six Lives: The Provision of Public Services to People with Learning Disabilities*. The Stationery Office, London.

Pointu A, Young J and Walsh K (2009) Improving health with acute liaison nursing. *Learning Disability Practice*, 12(5), 16–20.

Slevin E (2009) The importance of ethics. *Learning Disability Practice*, 12(3), 11.

The Rehabilitation of Offenders Act (1975) Exceptions Order. UK Act of Parliament.

The Safeguarding Vulnerable Groups Act (2006) UK Act of Parliament.

Thompson IE, Melia KM and Boyd KM (2000) *Nursing Ethics*, fourth edition. Churchill Livingstone, London.

UK Learning Disability Consultant Nurse Network (2006) *Shaping the Future: A Vision for Learning Disability Nursing*. UK Learning Disability Consultant Nurse Network, London, UK.

Whatt G (2008) Mental Capacity Act and Benevolent Deception under the Guise of 'Best Interests'. *Learning Disability Practice*, 11(3), 42–45 April 2008.

Wolfensberger W (1972) *The Principles of Normalisation in Human Management Services*. National Institute of Mental Retardation, Toronto.

Useful Websites and Contacts

ACCESSIBLE INFORMATION AND COMMUNICATION

Accessible Information
www.accessibility@mencap.org.uk

Communication Matters
www.communicationmatters.org.uk

Change Picture Bank
www.changepeople.co.uk

Easy Information
www.easyinfo.org.uk

Listening to patients
www.beingwithpatients@nhs.uk

Makaton
www.makaton.org

Signalong
www.signalong.org.uk

The Hospital Communication Book
www.communicationpeople.co.uk/Hospital%20Book.htm

Royal National Institute for the Blind Accessible Information
www.rnib.org.uk/access/

ADVOCACY AND SELF-HELP ORGANISATIONS

Central England People First
www.peoplefirst.org.uk

Disability Rights Commission
www.drc-gb.org

People First (National)
www.peoplefirstltd.com

General Hospital Care for People with Learning Disabilities, *First Edition* by Lynn Hannon and Julie Clift
© 2011 Blackwell Publishing Ltd

ISSUES AROUND AGEING

Age Concern England
www.ace.org.uk/

AUTISTIC SPECTRUM DISORDERS

Asperger's Syndrome
www.aspergersyndrome.co.uk

National Autistic Society (UK)
www.nas.org.uk

BRAIN INJURY

British Institute for Brain Injured Children
www.bibic.org.uk

CARERS

Caring About Carers
www.carers.gov.uk

Carers UK
www.carersonline.org.uk

Princess Royal Trust for Carers
Have a chat room where you can talk with other carers and a message board. People get together
    at 7 p.m. on the internet every evening. Tel: 020 7480 7788
www.carersonline.org

CEREBRAL PALSY

Scope
www.scope.org.uk/

CHALLENGING BEHAVIOUR

Challenging Behaviour Foundation
www.thecbf.org.uk

CHILDREN'S ISSUES

Childline
www.childline.org.uk

NSPCC
www.nspcc.org.uk

CONTINENCE

Association for Continence Advice
www.aca.uk.com

DISABILITY – GENERAL

Disability Alliance
www.disabilityalliance.org

Disability Now
www.disabilitynow.org.uk

Disabled Living Foundation
www.dlf.org.uk

Dyspraxia Foundation
www.dyspraxiafoundation.org.uk

The Family Fund
www.familyfund.org.uk

Joseph Rowntree Foundation
www.jrf.co.uk

Learning Disabilities
www.learningdisability.co.uk

Learning Disabilities Links
www.rnld.co.uk

National Institute of Neurological Disorders and Stroke (NINDS)
www.ninds.nih.gov/disorders

Norah Fry Research Centre
www.bris.ac.uk/Depts/NorahFry

Rett Syndrome Association UK
www.rettsyndrome.org.uk

EPILEPSY

British Epilepsy Association
www.epilepsy.org.uk
epilepsy@epilepsy.org.uk

Epilepsy Action (British Epilepsy Association)
www.epilepsy.org.uk

Lennox-Gastaut Support Group
Contact Andrew Gibson
GIBBO1@lennox-gastaut.frewwserve.co.uk

GOVERNMENT DEPARTMENTS

Department of Health
www.doh.gov.uk

Valuing People
www.valuingpeople.gov.uk

HEALTH ISSUES FOR PEOPLE WITH LEARNING DISABILITIES

Elfrida Society
www.elfrida.com

Intellectual Disability Health Information
www.intellectualdisability.info

HUMAN RIGHTS

Human Rights Act 1998
www.hmso.gov.uk/acts/acts1998/19980042.htm

Scottish Human Rights Centre
www.scottishhumanrightscentre.org.uk

LEARNING DISABILITY GENERAL

British Institute of Learning Disabilities
www.bild.org.uk/

Estia Centre
www.estiacentre.org

Foundation for People with Learning Disabilities
www.learningdisabilities.org.uk

Joseph Rowntree Foundation
www.jrf.org.uk

Mencap
www.mencap.org.uk

Learning Disabilities UK
www.learningdisabilitiesuk.org.uk

MEDICAL ISSUES

British Medical Association
www.bma.org.uk

MENTAL HEALTH ISSUES

Mental Health Care
www.mentalhealthcare.org

Mind
www.mind.org.uk/

MENTAL HEALTH ACT

Mental Health Act Commission
www.mhac.trent.nhs.uk

Mental Health Act Guide
www.hyperguide.co.uk/mha/

MENTAL HEALTH IN LEARNING DISABILITY

Institute for Dual Diagnosis
www.npi.ucla.ed/mhdd

PSYCHOLOGY

British Association for Behavioural and Cognitive Psychotherapies
www.babcp.org.uk

British Association for Counselling and Psychotherapy
www.counselling.co.uk

Cognitive-Behavioural Therapy
www.cognitivetherapy.com

SENSORY IMPAIRMENTS

Royal National Institute for Deaf People
www.rnid.org.uk

Royal National Institute of the Blind
www.rnib.org

SENSE
www.sense.org.uk

SPEECH AND LANGUAGE THERAPY

Royal College of Speech and Language Therapists
www.rcsit.org

SOCIAL WORK

British Association of Social Workers
www.basw.co.uk

SYNDROMES

Advice on Specific Conditions and Rare Disorders
www.cafamily.org.uk

Angelman's Syndrome
www.asclepius.com/angel

Birth Defects Foundation
www.birthdefects.co.uk

Cornelia de Lange Syndrome
www.cdls.org.uk

Down's Syndrome Association (UK)
www.dsa-uk.com

Down's Syndrome Association (USA)
http://nas.com/downsyn/index.html

Dysmorphic Syndromes
www.hgmp.mrc.ac.uk/DHMHD/view_human.html

Foetal Alcohol Syndrome (FAS)
To find out more, contact Margaret Murch
Margiemurch@blueyonder.co.uk

Fragile X Research Foundation
www.fraxa.org

Fragile X Society
www.fragilex.org.uk

Genes and Disease
www.ncbi.nih.gov/disease

Klinefelter's Syndrome
www.ksa-uk.co.uk

Prada Willi Association (UK)
www.pwsa-uk.demon.uk

Prada Willi Association USA
www.pwsausa.org

Rare Genetic Diseases in Children
www.med.nyu.edu/rgdc/homenew.htm

Rett's Syndrome Association (UK)
www.rettsyndrome.org.uk

Smith–Magenis Syndrome
www.kumc.edc/gec/support/smith-ma.html

Tourette's Syndrome
www.tsa.org.uk

Tuberous Sclerosis Association
www.tuberous-sclerosis.org

Turner's Syndrome UK
www.tss.org.uk

Turner's Syndrome (USA)
www.turner-syndrome-us.org

UK Resources for Down's Syndrome
www.43green.freeserve.co.uk/uk downs syndrome/ukdsinfo.html

Williams Syndrome
www.williams-syndrome.org.uk

Index

triage, 43, 70, 73
  National Triage Scale, 43
Trust Boards, 24

undiagnosed conditions, 14, 21
under-protection, 98
underweight, 19
unemployment, 16
unhealthy lifestyles, 19

values and beliefs, 170, 186, 202, 214–17
Valuing People, 3, 22, 33, 118, 219–20
verbal information, 88
verbal prompts, 143

Vetting and Barring Scheme, 211–14
  regulated activity, 212
  controlled activity, 212
video, 93
visiting hours, 23
visual impairment, 9, 19, 111
vulnerability in hospital, 20, 35, 40

waiting time, 27, 29, 45–7, 73, 88
Walker Warburg Syndrome, 227
withholding information, 202–5
withholding treatment, 169, 186–8
World Health Organisation (WHO), 3

x-ray, 28